The Sevenfold Circle
Self Awareness in Dance

Lynn Frances
and
Richard Bryant-Jefferies

To Helen
Dance on in joy
With our love

Lynn & Richard

FINDHORN
Press

First published 1998

ISBN 1 899171 37 1

British Library Cataloguing-in-Publication Data.
A catalogue record for this book is available from the British Library.

Cover design and book layout by Findhorn Press
'Self Awareness in Dance' logo © 1996 Lynn Frances & Richard Bryant-Jefferies
Printed and bound WSOY, Finland

Published by
Findhorn Press
The Park, Findhorn, Forres IV36 0TZ, Scotland
tel +44 (0)1309 690582 • fax 690036
email thierry@findhorn.org
http://www.findhorn.org/findhornpress/

Contents

Introduction 5

Acknowledgements 8

Part 1 — Two Paths One Goal 9
A Journey of Self-Discovery 10
My Voyage of Rediscovery 21
Working Together 31

Part 2 — Sacred Circle Dance 39
Origins of Sacred Circle Dance 40
Sacred Space —Walls do have Ears 42
Sacred Dance and Spirituality 47
Symbolism in the Circle 53
International Language of Dance 58
Getting to Know Other Cultures 64

Part 3 — The Seven Rays 75
A Sevenfold View of Life 76
Reflections on the Life-cycle 85
Colouring Psychological Growth 97
Shaping the Nations of the World 102
Call to Love 110

Part 4 — Collaboration — the Workshops 113
Dancing the Sevenfold Energies of Life 114
Dancing the Zodiac: the Soul's Journey to Greater Light 122
A Little Smackerel of Something 142
The Cross and the Circle: Living Symbols 152
Beyond Balance — Towards Complementarity 165
Celebrating the Spirit in a Material World 175

Transition from the Old to the New 189
From the Love of Power to the Power of Love 200
Epilogue 213

Appendices 215
Reflections for the Future 215
Unity in Diversity Teambuilding 223

Index 230

Introduction

From conception...

We were in Poland when we decided to write this book. We had been invited over there to lead workshops at two summer camps in 1996. We were in the mountains in the south of the country right on the Slovak border. The river marking the boundary between the two countries flowed gently past us as we sat on its bank in the summer sunshine. We were very relaxed: it was our third visit and it was a great thrill to be back in the company of friends old and new — we feel quite at home in Poland, we call it our second home. We had a little time to ourselves and the book was conceived.

It was our second day and we had ambled down to the water from the hostel, where the camp was being held, talking of this and that. The flowers were beautiful on the roadside verges; the peacock butterflies were in profusion on the hemp agrimony; and we recognised many of the flowers and trees: Nature does not know the artificial boundaries we create round ourselves and our countries. It was hard to believe that just the other side of the river was Slovakia, where the people speak a different language. They looked the same as us as they walked along the path on 'their' side.

We sat and mused, threw stones into the water, watched as twigs that we lobbed in were taken by the current. We allowed ourselves to be taken by the current of our separate and mutual thoughts.

"I think we should write a book, you know," said Richard as he tried to skim a flat stone across the water somewhat unsuccessfully.

"Mm," responded Lynn, paying more attention to her twig, which had just got caught on a branch in the river.

A few moments passed. "Are you serious?" Lynn questioned.

"Why not?" replied Richard idly throwing in another stick.

"What about?"

Richard hesitated momentarily while he collected his thoughts.

"Circle Dance and the Seven Rays for a start."

"But how can we bring them together in one book?"

"Well we bring them together in a workshop. That's a start."

"And we've already been writing articles about it, haven't we?" Lynn was gaining enthusiasm now.

"I know how we could do it. You write about Sacred Circle Dance and I'll do the Seven Rays."

"And why not write about all the other workshops too."

In a few minutes we were fired with enthusiasm and had an outline structure. We even had in mind potential reviewers of the finished product! Well, you have to dream, otherwise nothing ever comes to pass.

So that is what happens when we are away from the hustle and bustle of everyday life. The impossible suddenly becomes not only possible but a living entity. The book gained an energy of its own and every experience became a potential anecdote. We had to mull it over for another two weeks before we could sit down in front of the computer and put our thoughts onto paper (or screen). Nevertheless, the seed was germinating and by the time we arrived home the shoot was forcing its way through the concrete of our thoughts of "No I can't", "Nobody will ever read it" and "Who will publish it?", to emerge triumphant. We had to write. It was compelling and demanding.

...to birth...

At first sight it seems that Sacred Circle Dance and the Seven Rays are an unlikely combination of subjects for a book. However, it is precisely these two topics which brought us together in the first place, as we will describe in the following pages. Our two journeys in life had taken us on quite different paths, yet unknown to us these paths were to converge in a totally unexpected and unplanned way.

We brought our individual knowledge and skills into a relationship which subsequently led us both into a new and shared direction. Sacred Circle Dance is an expression of life, of human relationships and our interaction with the world around us. The Seven Rays is a model through which we can understand ourselves, each other and our communities. Together they give us an opportunity for self-investigation in a safe and supportive environment free of associations with the hectic round of daily life.

Both of these topics may be new to you. We hope that when you reach the end of this book you will understand what we are bringing together and will want to explore our approach in more depth. We hope to fire you with curiosity.

You will see that the original idea of dancing the Seven Rays has led us to many other themes. The *creativity* of giving birth to these 'babies' has been a wonderfully inspiring and instructive process. Together we have discovered that creativity is a fundamental force of life, and that the greatest block to this tendency lies in believing that we are not creative. If either of us feels that we cannot do something, we ask ourselves: what is the origin of this disbelief in my potential? Is it based on a genuine experience or, as is so often the case, some negative self-perception, the result of a 'put-down' by somebody way back in my past?

One example of this occurs in nearly every workshop that we run. Somebody believes that they cannot dance. By the end of a day they know they can, and a new phase of life and expression has begun. This is a source of constant joy and excitement to us, to see these miracles happening before our very eyes.

For some people there is something inherently alien about the idea of community dance, yet in many cultures it is as natural as walking. There is nothing fundamentally difficult about it, but our mind-set may stop us enjoying our body's movement and beauty in motion. As you will see in the following pages it can be more revealing to go wrong in a dance than to do it perfectly: even 'mistakes' are honoured and welcomed in our workshops!

In many traditions dance has been used to help people to experience themselves and even to enter into mystical and/or ecstatic states. Has this approach to dance been lost? Maybe, and yet for many young people in the West the current dance scene, whilst intensely individualistic, contains an urge to achieve a heightened sense of self awareness. How much more might be gained from dancing together in circles. The greatest 'high' is the quality of the human relationships that make the dance possible.

We would like to say a word of appreciation to each other. We have each sparked off in the other something that we did not believe was there. We have drawn each other out, we have discovered hidden depths and heights. We have created something beautiful in our work together, that is truly borne out of relationship. It demonstrates for us the old maxim that 'the whole is greater than the sum of the parts'. Neither of us would have done this alone.

Finally, none of our workshops would have been possible without the participation of those of you who have shared the dance with us. Our biggest "thank you" has to go to you.

...and realisation!

Lynn and Richard
Summer 1997

Acknowledgements

Special thanks to Annie König for her editorial persistence and her belief in what we are doing.

We are very grateful to Laura Shannon, Tricia Elsey and Jane Baker for their helpful and encouraging comments on an early draft of selected chapters.

We would like to thank Keith Ruffell for the wonderful photographs he took of Sacred Circle Dance, and for dancing with us afterwards.

Last, but by no means least, we would like to say a big "thank you!" to Diana Mills for her continued support and encouragement.

We would also like to acknowledge the following publications:

The Review (now *Science of Thought Review*) in which part of the chapter on "Sacred Dance and Spirituality" first appeared.

Christian in which part of the chapter on "Sacred Dance and Spirituality" first appeared.

Journal of Esoteric Psychology in which a version of the chapter "Reflections on the Life-cycle" appeared.

Part 1

Two Paths One Goal

by Lynn and Richard

*We each had to have trodden
our own individual paths
to a particular point
before we were in a certain sense
ready to begin to journey together.*

A Journey of Self-discovery

Lynn

When I first came across Sacred Circle Dance in 1982, I was immediately struck by the feeling of well-being that it generated. I had never felt so at peace with the world and myself. Even now, after all these years, people tell me I change when I dance, and I can certainly feel it within me — I flow, I am graceful, and I am full of joy. This is not just a 'quick fix' when I am dancing: the way I dress has changed dramatically, from sombre brown and grey suits and trousers to hide behind, to brightly coloured clothes that show I am pleased to be seen!

As a teenager I went to a dance practically every Saturday evening: in those days and with those friends, ballroom dancing was a natural part of life. It was the way we socialised and the way we met other people. If it was not a full blown dance it was Scottish Country Dancing and we had a wonderful time. Gradually I lost touch with that group when I went to college, and I found to my astonishment and dismay that very few of my new 'crowd' could dance. The men in particular were most reluctant to take the floor; when they did they usually managed to do a waltz with four beats to the bar! It seemed unlikely that I would ever whirl round a dance floor again.

Life went on and I had not realised how much I missed the exercise and the exhilaration until I finally encountered Sacred Circle Dance. Here was a form of dance which did not need a partner, yet I still had contact with others, which is a very important aspect for me — I do not really like the modern dancing in which people dance on their own and nobody cares whether there is anyone else there or not.

At last I could dance again and I felt wonderful, but there was one drawback. At the time I had bad back trouble. I had spent many weeks over the previous few years flat on my back unable to do anything except feel sorry for myself. It was a miracle that I could dance at all. At first I could only do a couple of dances and then I had to sit out with my back against a wall (this is difficult in a marquee, where I first danced, so it had to be flat on the ground!). Nevertheless the feeling that I had after dancing was one I wanted more of: the exhilaration; the peace; the companionship; the joy. The problems with my back seemed less important; I had to dance.

A spiritual quest

I was brought up as a Presbyterian, and as a teenager and young adult I went to church every week and attended the youth club. It was my life. I then found myself with a whole host of doubts. I began to see life in a subtly different way which is very difficult to describe. It was a traumatic time because I was questioning the beliefs of a lifetime and yet I wanted a broader outlook on life. I wanted to be able to embrace ideas other than those of the church.

I finally made the break amidst considerable self-doubt and anguish within my family. I then discovered the spirituality/psychology section in the local library and started reading avidly. I had started my real spiritual journey: I was beginning to find myself and what I truly believed. A few books stand out from this period. *The Magic of Findhorn* by Paul Hawken[1] made a deep impression on me with its wonderful story of hardship and unforeseen circumstances leading to the creation of a spiritual community. Could this be the way life was? Are we led to our true mission if we can only stop trying to control our lives for long enough to hear and acknowledge the signs?

The Yogi Ramacharaka books[2] *Fourteen Lessons in Yogi Philosophy and Oriental Occultism*, the *Advanced Course* and *The Hindu Science of Breath* came at one of the times when I was on my back in agony. I remember really working with the lessons and beginning to use visualisation techniques to heal myself. By this time I had taken up Yoga and found it to be a wonderful way of exercising and relaxing. The philosophy behind it fascinated me too and I was learning more about the eastern way of life.

I began to find that I *understood* aspects of life: I *knew* rather than believed. This was a revelation. It was also surprising to me that nothing I was doing was in conflict with the teachings of Christ with which I had been brought up. In fact quite the opposite: it was all part and parcel of the same search for truth. I saw the teachings of the Bible in a different light: no longer was my belief system founded on fear and guilt but on a real relationship with the spiritual. Indeed it was not a 'belief' system but a 'knowledge' system. I was on a glorious journey which might take me anywhere, and anywhere it took me was where I should be!

My journey led me to meditation: I had seen notices locally about classes in someone's home, but had not had the courage to go along. Then I saw it in the adult education brochure and it felt safe to join! It will be no surprise to you that it was the same people leading it as had been advertising on the notice boards. This later proved to be another

---

1.   Published by Souvenir Press. (Out of print.)
2.   Published by L N Fowler and Co Ltd, Romford, UK.

turning point in my life.

Alongside this spiritual quest, my formal education and career had followed a scientific route. After gaining a degree in Mathematics and Physics at Kings College, London I went into computing as a Trainee Programmer with Elliott Medical Automation. Here I learned the basics of programming and by the time I left was helping to run courses for medical personnel. Over a period of 15 years with a number of different companies, I worked my way up the computing ladder to become a Senior Project Leader in a large multinational firm selling agricultural chemicals.

Almost as soon as I started to meditate I decided to give up my job. There were many reasons for my decision, but the strongest was my conscience: I could no longer support the use of dangerous chemicals when I was gardening organically. Life for me had to be more natural; I remain convinced that we are polluting the planet by our efforts to control nature. Meditation had somehow given me the strength to stand up for what I knew to be right. It was a hard decision, nevertheless, because I had reached a senior position and been promoted above some of my male colleagues. Was I letting down the whole of womankind? Should I have persevered, if only to prove that women *can* succeed in business? The winter of 1979/80 was a time of much heart-searching, yet now I have no regrets.

I remember Richard saying soon after we met, "I don't know what you do for a living apart from teaching Circle Dancing". "My 'other job' is as an editor for scientific journals and books." As I told him this, I had a very clear picture in my mind. I found myself telling him, "I see it as a cross; the editing keeps my mind active and my feet firmly on the ground; the dancing keeps my feet (and body) active and my head up in the clouds!" I thoroughly enjoy the contrast: it is stimulating and exciting.

Strange encounters

My first encounter with Sacred Circle Dance in 1982 was at a 'Green Gathering' near Glastonbury. It was a very strange experience for me because it came at the end of a four-month trip round the British Isles in a motor caravan with only two companions and one of them was a dog! Suddenly I was surrounded by about 3000 other people camping in close proximity. It was a great shock to the system and my defence was to keep myself to myself and not partake in anything that was happening.

Then I heard there was something called Sacred Dance being held every morning and evening. It was my salvation then and ever since.

I nearly gave up after the second dance because I found it so difficult: I felt I was never going to master it, and this was presumably the next-to-easiest dance. Fortunately we were there for a week and I was inevitably and irrecoverably drawn to dance at each session. I mastered dance number two and many more during that time.

By the end of the week I was well and truly hooked. I frantically made enquiries about dancing near my home, but it seemed there was none within easy reach. That was how it was in the early days — dance groups were few and far between. However, there was to be a day workshop the following weekend not too far away, assuming we arrived home in time and did not prolong our travels.

That Saturday in August found me dancing outside at Moorhurst in Dorking, Surrey which was then being run as a centre for all manner of alternative activities. I had a wonderful day and was even more determined to continue to dance. The teacher from the Green Gathering was at that day and announced that she was going to take the dance 'on tour'. I immediately started thinking about the possibility of arranging for her to do a day near me and getting some of my friends to come along to share the experience. The negotiations all fell through though, because it seemed impossible to organise a mutually convenient date. My dancing days looked like being over yet again.

Coincidence

At that time I had little experience of the concept that nothing happens by chance, that 'co-incidence' is just that — two things occurring at the same time. This was the beginning of a new phase in my journey of self-discovery and understanding of the laws of the universe.

The next year in May I went to a day put on by my Yoga teacher. I had not danced for nearly nine months. Perhaps I had almost forgotten about it and yet I guess I had not. On the programme for the day was a speaker who let us down at the eleventh hour; I cannot even remember now what he/she was supposed to be talking about. My teacher was a very persuasive person and had managed to find a substitute speaker to talk about Esoteric Healing. So, after the morning of Yoga exercises, we sat down to listen to a most interesting talk by Dinah Lawson, who has since become a firm friend.

Right at the end, almost as an afterthought, she mentioned that she was involved with organising solstice and equinox festivals in Hampshire and would leave some leaflets out in case anyone was interested. I took one and it sounded like my sort of day: a pilgrimage up Old

Winchester Hill in the morning followed by a celebration in a nearby hall in the afternoon, including Sacred Dance. So the summer solstice saw me in East Meon village hall and I was dancing again!

Michael Loxton, who led the dance that day, had been at Moorhurst the previous year (another 'coincidence') and I found that he ran a class about 30 miles from home. The next evening I went along and that was the start of six happy years of dancing regularly at Washington in West Sussex. (The group still runs there under different leadership but I have moved even further away now.)

At the time I was completely taken aback by the set of circumstances that had brought me and Sacred Dance back together again. It was the beginning of a period of great change in my life: new friends; new self-image; greater understanding of myself; more self-confidence; and a deeper connection with my spirituality. Two or three years later would see me leading the dancing at these same solstice and equinox festivals, but what about the interim?

My first group

After a few weeks of attending the group in Washington, I decided that it was not enough! I had to dance more often; I had to pass on my enjoyment to others. So I invited about twenty people to supper. Little did they know they would be expected to dance! I had bought the only four tapes of music that were available at the time. I learnt three dances well enough to teach — the really simple ones.

I made everyone dance for their supper! "Before we eat we're all going to dance": to me I sounded a bit scared! Well, it was a nerve-wracking experience that first time. I had practised and practised those three dances until the carpet started to look worn. I was terrified that I would forget the steps and/or people would think I was crazy — or, worse still, not like the dances. The actual instructing was not too much of a problem as my previous career in computing had involved a fair amount of lecturing and teaching. I guess it was that the dances were so important to me and it was crucial that they were well received.

It helped that we were able to dance outside, because that seems to increase the magic of the atmosphere that is created. Everyone joined in and after my three dances my guests were demanding, "Let's do some more!" "But I only know those three," I admitted. "OK, we'll do those again then." "Right, we'll have supper first, and then dance in the moonlight." And so it was. We danced again and I had the core of my first dance group.

We started meeting monthly at my house on a Sunday afternoon until the autumn weather beat us. Then I hired the local village hall and people paid a contribution towards the costs. At first the numbers were small but that was an advantage for me as a novice. I could just about keep ahead of them and introduce one new dance each time. After each session I felt wonderful: this was me!

One thing I discovered in those early days was how to make a mistake! There were many as you might expect, but I have always been a bit of a perfectionist and it was really hard for me to get it wrong. There was the classic occasion when I did a dance at entirely the wrong speed; and the time I had to give up trying to teach one of them because I simply could not get it right. Over the years I have learnt how to do this gracefully and to laugh at my own mistakes, but in those days I was devastated. My journey of self-discovery was teaching me new lessons.

I remember the first time Michael came to my class. I even asked him, "Do you want to lead it?" His reply was, "No, thank you. I want to dance in someone else's circle". At the time I was rather taken aback and very nervous. Now I entirely understand: I too find it important to be on the receiving end sometimes rather than always being 'centre stage'. When I look back, I realise that I was heavily conditioned into thinking that 'teacher' must be much better than me and would not want to be taught by me. A new dimension emerged for me, and a new confidence in my own ability.

New developments

A year later found me leading my first day workshop. What a lesson that was! In fact it was more a lesson in how not to do it that in how to do it! Far too many dances and far too little teaching; far too much that was new and far too little repetition. But that is the way to learn, and interestingly most of the people who attended that day in 1984 are still dancing today.

I then started two regular groups at Adult Education evening classes. This heralded another 'coincidence'. Never before had Circle Dance been on an evening class syllabus: quite independently, five or six of the ten or twelve people then teaching approached their local Adult Education Institutes and began groups in the same year! Once the thought was out on the 'air waves' it was picked up and acted on. I was beginning to discover the potential of group experience.

In those days we had to be quite careful about the title of a course. Yoga had finally become accepted as a suitable subject. Meditation was just becoming a regular feature of the programme. But 'sacred' was not a word that should appear. Hence we called it Circle Dance: what is lost in the name is certainly not lost in the experience. Sacred Circle Dance by any other name...

When I think about it now I realise that it was an amazing departure from my normal way of behaviour. In my career as a computer programmer and systems analyst I had been gently led into giving lectures and talks; I had enjoyed it in the end, but I had never before volunteered my services. In this instance I even had to exercise a certain amount of gentle persuasion! For the Heads of Adult Education it was a case of, "Well, I'll put it on the brochure and we'll see what happens, but I don't hold out much hope". In the event it went like a bomb and in the first term my classes easily reached the minimum number required.

So I was launched — or, perhaps, more importantly, I had launched myself.

Finding myself

My search for new dances to teach led me to workshops all over the South of England. I travelled miles to dance with other teachers. I collected dances avidly and felt it desperately important to pass them on to others. I wrote extensive notes and was adamant that the steps should be conveyed as accurately as was humanly possible.

I could begin to observe an obsession in myself. I guess we all have some form of obsession, more or less damaging. Over the years I have learnt that quantity is not essential; neither is novelty. In my experience people like to learn an occasional new dance, but the ones they really love are the 'golden oldies'. There is a familiarity about these dances that makes people feel comfortable: the body can move without interference from the head. When a new dance is introduced the initial learning is a mental activity. Later on the dancers can allow themselves to 'be danced', because the steps have been incorporated into the body.

This was a great lesson to me. When I came to this realisation it freed me from the pressure to teach ever new, ever more complex dances. All that did was to prove something about me: it did little to enhance the enjoyment or experience for others. What a revelation: I no longer had to be one step ahead (or one dance ahead). I was free of the old conditioning from back in my schooldays to excel.

To illustrate the sort of conditioning we are subjected to, here is a little anecdote about a children's group I ran some years ago. They were a lively bunch and kept me on my toes! They found some of the dances quite difficult, so when I taught them one that went really well I said, "That was great — let's do it again!". The immediate response was, "Why do it again if we did it right?". It opened my eyes to the mentality that our educational system encourages: if you cannot do it, work at it until you can; when you can do it, move on to the next thing. This allows no enjoyment in being able to do something well and chastises people if they cannot. So we all strive to be something we are not, thus concentrating on our weaknesses rather than our strengths. The work Richard and I are doing with dance uses the reverse philosophy by bringing out the strengths, but more of that later.

Gaining self esteem

After a particularly wonderful weekend of dancing with teachers in the South East of England, I realised that I could no longer continue in my 18-year marriage. For years it had been increasingly difficult for me and yet I believed that I had made a commitment for life. I carried on in great pain until that day when I suddenly felt strong enough to be able to say, "I don't need this any more". We had been for counselling, we had sought advice, but we had different ideas about what marriage meant and eventually the incompatibility became intolerable.

We had managed to keep a very good 'public image' so it was a great shock to many people: we both danced (and still do); we ran workshops together; but our relationship had fallen apart. At last I could say that I deserved better than that. I could even see that I was better off on my own — it took the dance to help me see my own qualities. The dance had brought me friends who valued me for what I am, made me understand my own abilities, required nothing of me; my self-esteem had improved; I valued myself.

It was an extremely traumatic time, but gradually people started saying that I was like a butterfly coming out of a chrysalis, or a plant beginning to blossom. I was finding a new 'me' unencumbered by anyone else's requirements; at last I had time to discover my true potential. Dancing, and particularly my regular groups, kept me going in those early days of being on my own; it was my lifeline, giving me a social life and an income! Sacred Circle Dance has an amazing ability to make me feel whole, to give me strength and the courage to cope with the stresses of life. I can go to a class feeling tired, emotionally drained or even ill: I leave feeling elated, energised and fit for anything!

Developing the dance

For the first time I started running workshops on my own and they went really well. We celebrated the Celtic festivals in dance, we danced a folk tale, the seasons of the year, a rainbow, the life cycle, the labyrinth and magic circle references in Shakespeare's *Tempest*, the signs of the zodiac, masculine and feminine. The list grew and grew and my use of the dance became more orientated towards helping people to experience something about themselves and the world around them. I realised that the dances held a key to self-discovery: it seemed that the rhythmic movement in a group of like-minded people became more than the dance. In my workshops I began to use it as a form of expression to link us with our essence, our inner being.

So now the dances become more than just physical movement, the dance begins to live. Participants feel the energy, the emotion; concepts are no longer something intangible but a direct experience.

I was so excited about this use of the dance. It was only later that I realised that this was really taking them back to their roots in the rhythm of community life.

I attempt to teach the dances as accurately as I know how, but the emphasis is on moving round the circle together. Whether individual people are doing the 'right' steps in the 'right' way is less important than the feeling that is generated. However, I will go over a dance until the majority of participants have mastered the steps: this enhances the feeling of togetherness. The flow of the circle improves and the full benefit of the dance is realised when we are working in harmony. That is an interesting word, 'harmony'. In modern usage it seems to have degenerated into meaning all doing the same. In music it means all doing something different and there lies the beauty! So it is with dance: we each bring our own expression, our own character to the movements.

Another turning point

By now my life had become a search after truth. I had read numerous books, assimilated other people's views of life, but this was not enough. I had to know for myself, have my own ideas. I went through periods of intense reading, followed inevitably by a sort of 'burn out' during which I simply did not want to see another book. I began to realise that it was these periods that became my growth times. It was not absorbing the philosophies of other people that for me led to greatest spiritual development but looking inside me and finding *my* truth.

My quest led me, after a great deal of Soul-searching, to go on a course given by Michelle Vezeau from Canada entitled 'Learning to Channel'. I had heard Michelle speak the previous year, but I had felt no great urge to attend her course. In fact I held (and still do hold) a rather cynical view of channelling. There seems to me to be a lot of 'hype' involved that I find extremely off-putting. I remain wary of it, especially when personally I feel that outrageous claims are made about the origins of the material and its import.

However, I found myself irresistibly drawn to the course Michelle ran in the UK in 1990. It was totally absorbing and it turned out to be another turning point in my search for truth. Over the weekend we were taught to channel what Michelle calls Source. After all, she said, if we have a connection to Source why not tap it — it all made perfect sense. I could relate to that much better than the idea of channelling discarnate entities, which had always been a concern to me. This was not to be trance channelling either: we simply went into our hearts and sought the answers within ourselves.

At the end of the weekend I was still sceptical, particularly about my own abilities. Yet over the next few weeks I found myself writing pieces that I would never have written before; there were certain characteristics which seemed to be significant, such as a lot of alliteration, repetition of words (which I had been taught at a very early age was bad style!), and even the use of words that I had to look up in the dictionary to check their meaning (and they were always perfect in the context!).

I persevered. I asked questions about the structure of the universe; the nature of time; and things of concern in my personal life. I received answers and they helped me to understand. I have continued with the practice: that is how I think of it, because anything that is worthwhile needs to be worked at. It is much like meditation in that respect.

I believe that I am tapping the depths of my being. It is the Source of great wisdom — the result of many incarnations in this world and my interconnectedness with everything. Within me I have infinite knowledge, boundless wisdom: I cannot link to it all at the moment; that would probably blow my mind. Yet gradually new revelations are made: it is as if the doors are opening to new chambers of my being and I am aware of another level of understanding.

It is very exciting, although I have found it difficult to write about. It is something like trying to express my personal feelings towards Sacred Circle Dancing: I cannot find the words that will tell you the wonder of it — perhaps both these aspects of my life, that are so important to me, defy words. There is nothing to take the place of individual experience, and I come round again to needing to know my own truth!

Healing properties

What of my back? Even while writing this I have been so excited about Sacred Circle Dance and my own journey that I have forgotten to mention my back! That was how it was: suddenly it was no longer a problem. It started to improve as soon as I started dancing: it began to strengthen; I could dance for longer without pain; I could forget it while I danced. Of course there were a few lapses, including the memorable occasion when I watched a workshop from the sidelines! This was very frustrating but when I first started dancing I would never have imagined that I could have run a day, let alone make it part of my life's work.

Over the last eight years I have had virtually no trouble. There has been the occasional twinge and a few visits to a remedial masseur but my previous problems have dissolved. I put it down to dance. I do not know whether it is because the dance has become so important to me and nothing, not even my back, is going to stop me, or whether my body has healed as a result of the dancing. Perhaps it is a combination of the two. I do not really need to know the ins and outs: it is better and that is enough for me.

The next chapter

The period of five years when I lived on my own was a time of great personal growth. From hating to be in my flat alone in the evening in the early days, it gradually became a haven to escape to. I liked being able to make my own decisions: I was not answerable to anyone. Then for the first time I spent one weekend entirely on my own, no visitors, just me in my own space: I loved it! The next week I met Richard!

My Voyage of Rediscovery

Richard

It is strange where life takes you — if you let it! I certainly never expected to be involved in running dance workshops. My memories of dancing are of rather frenetic movement at the local youth club disco which were brought to an inevitable and sudden halt only when I fell off my platform soles! Mind you, I had by then begun reading books on spiritual growth and eastern philosophy and I guess somewhere in the back of my mind I had a sense that life was a dance. I just had not found my own music — or my own steps.

As a teenager I began buying second-hand books on mysticism and esoteric philosophy. I was encouraged by my parents who were themselves seeking answers to questions in their own lives. I remember my father coming home one evening with two volumes of Madame Blavatsky's *The Secret Doctrine* on his Honda 50 — one volume in each back pannier. We all struggled to understand the wisdom of those two books; however, as I like to think looking back, they at least provided excellent stability in a cross wind!

For me there is a deep esoteric truth here in that we do need some kind of stabilising factor in our lives, something that we can grow our roots into. I like the image of the tree, standing proud and upright, rooted firmly in Mother Earth and able to bend with the breeze. It has a power and a majesty. Whilst we need to be open-minded, we also need to have something solid. It is all too easy to flit from one idea to the next, absorbing everything regardless of what it is, and without really thinking things through for ourselves to enable us to develop our own philosophy of life, the universe and everything. This philosophical model or pattern of thinking we then use to measure our experiences and to choose what we may need to add to our understanding, and what may now need to be left behind.

Going back to my teenage years, the books I read sowed a lot of seeds in my own mind as I wrestled to grasp the nature of the Law of Karma and the idea of cosmic evolution. It all made sense somehow and yet my mind was stretched to the edge of its comprehension. It felt as though I was reminding myself of things that I already knew.

Indeed, looking back, my whole life has been like this — not a voyage of discovery, but of rediscovery. I remain convinced that my Soul is my true essence and being, and that my normal consciousness is a spark involved in the experience of matter and separation. Therefore something in me knows more than I am presently conscious of. I want to find what I already 'know'. In my work (both as a counsellor/therapist and with the *Self Awareness in Dance* workshops) I am trying to help other people on a similar journey.

First steps

I used to visit a wonderful old mill in Norfolk — Itteringham Mill — owned at that time by the mystic and poet Derek Neville. Here I was in my element, sitting in dusty rooms and corridors pouring over ancient (and some not so ancient) tomes. It was there that I bought a rather faded blue book, and as I write this now I feel the tears welling up in my eyes. It was the start of a journey and a relationship which remains with me today. The book was entitled, *Letters on Occult Meditation*, written by Alice Bailey — to this day the only first edition of her writings that I have. Something in me was coming home, though I did not know it then.

Why I bought the book, who knows. It was an old dusty tome, somewhat frayed around the edges, and I did not understand it. Nevertheless, something prompted me and I took it home; it sat on the shelf for at least two years before I finally read it. So often this happens. There is a connectedness that bridges time into the future, pressing us to obtain today what is required tomorrow, although at the time we do not appreciate its significance. Have you ever picked up a book sometime after acquiring it and found yourself thinking, yes, now I know why I bought this one?

Books have always been important to me. If I visit someone's home and I see no books it feels as though there is something missing. As I sit here now looking at the bookshelves in my study, I am reminded of an archaeological dig. You know how the archaeologist digs down through the layers to uncover periods of history? My bookshelves are like that. There is the early, mystical phase of Joel Goldsmith leading to my first exploration of eastern philosophy with Yogi Ramacharaka. There are a number of publications from The Theosophical Society, including titles by Madame Blavatsky and Annie Besant, which led to the appearance on the shelves of the Alice Bailey books. There then followed a variety of encounters, including: the scientific–mystical world-view of Teilhard de Chardin; Krishnamurti; the psychological theories of Carl Jung; David Spangler and the 'New Age' movement; Thomas Paine whose political, social and economic writings remain close to my heart; Ralph Waldo Emerson; and more recently the work of Carl Rogers.

Acquiring my first Alice Bailey book, however, did seem to be a turning point. The next 20 years became a time of exploration, and self-exploration; for much of that period her writings have been my map and my compass. It was through her philosophy that I was introduced to the Seven Rays, that magnificent concept of creation having a sevenfold nature within which we each live and move and have our being.

My mind and heart opened to many other important concepts. Probably of greatest significance has been the idea of conscious evolution — that there are cosmic laws driving evolution forward, in particular those of cause and effect (karma) and rebirth. As a child I can remember one night feeling overwhelmed by the sense of the infinity of creation — the immensity of the idea that there was no end, simply continuity through æons of time. It seemed to stretch ahead beyond the limit of my mind to comprehend. It seemed awesome. I suppose it was the stirring of a faint memory of how I knew it to be, yet as a child, no longer conscious of my connection with the immortal Soul-aspect of my nature, it did seem very scary.

I remember, too, as a teenager writing an essay at school on 'The Mind'. I described the ideas from eastern philosophy concerning karma, rebirth, the concept of planes of being, prana and the etheric body. We had been given free rein to choose our own topic, and this was what was holding my interest at the time. I still wonder what the teacher really made of it. I got 20 out of 20 for it so I guess it must have made some impact!

During the late 1970s I joined the Arcane School, originally founded by Alice Bailey in the 1920s. This gave me a focus for my development and further exploration of her writings. The School requires students to undertake daily meditation, regular study and to develop a life of service. These form a fundamental triplicity that lie at the heart of spiritual growth.

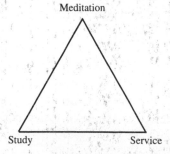

Meditation

Figure 1.
A triangle for spiritual growth

Study   Service

The idea is that through meditation we can cultivate inner, conscious sensitivity to deeper realms of being via the Soul or spiritual Self. Spiritual study focuses our minds and provides a way to refine our thought processes. In a sense, the mind is formed of subtle matter and, as we seek in meditation to resonate to subtle emanations from spiritual realms, we need a mind that is sensitive and inclusive enough to be able to grasp what is registered with clarity and with the minimum of distortion. Knowledge and insight carries with it responsibility — the responsibility of applying within the sphere of our daily life what we now know. It is important that all three are present. Then, inspiration can flow through into the mind to be grasped and applied in the routine of daily living through service. Service is the natural effect of developing contact with the Soul, indeed it is the manner in which the Soul expresses itself within humanity.

The Arcane School has been right for me. These days there are so many choices for people seeking to develop a deeper understanding of themselves and it can be hard to know where to begin. As with all philosophies you need to learn the language and the terminology but persistence will bear fruit. Do not expect spiritual growth to be a rosy experience of light, love and harmony. It is far more likely that all hell breaks loose as you are forced by your own process of growth to face up to the limitations, the tendencies towards separateness and selfishness, lodged within your nature. Yes, we want to enter into greater light so that we might then carry that light into the world, but we have to dissipate the blocks that obscure the light. It is well said that at every turn of the path we meet ourselves coming the other way and obstructing our progress. Patterns that have been established over many lives need facing, acknowledging and uprooting.

I do not intend to put people off, for to tread the spiritual path in life is the only true way to live. If you feel the urge to engage more fully with the spiritual Self you will be undaunted by the struggle because something in you will know that nothing else matters. The spark of consciousness that you are has heard the call of the Soul, the flame, from which it originated, and the power that draws the spark back to the flame is the most powerful force in creation — Love.

The Lucis Trust

In the mid-1980s I was invited to work at the Lucis Trust, the organisation established by Alice Bailey as a vehicle for her work: it was a time for me to absorb the ideas contained within her spiritual philosophy even more intensely. It brought me many wonderful experiences and a real opportunity to meet interesting people and to learn about the tremendous range of leading-edge projects and ideas being formulated around the world.

One of my jobs was to scan incoming material for information that might be used in Lucis Trust publications. It enabled me to see something of the planet-wide process taking place as individuals and groups seek to pioneer new ideas and possible solutions to world problems. It felt like being part of a global meditation, so many people directing the power of their hearts and minds towards lifting the human condition and helping us to reconnect with our spiritual roots. From the huge, international non-governmental organisations (NGOs) to the local, community-based organisations (CBOs) there exists a chain of service on our planet that holds the key to our collective future. There is no excuse for non-participation any more. Everywhere there is human need, and everywhere there are groups and individuals seeking to help meet that need.

I think back to that phase of my life and two occasions more than any other touch me deeply. The first was when I was chairing a session of the World Goodwill[3] seminar in London and the speaker was Professor James Lovelock — a wonderful, visionary thinker. The session went well and passed off without incident. However, over the coming weeks a strange experience occurred. I found my mind somehow sharpened in a way that I cannot describe in words. I was spending evenings reading *The Secret Doctrine* and Alice Bailey's *A Treatise on Cosmic Fire* as if my mind was a sponge. It was as though my mental energy body had been stimulated into heightened activity and, looking back, I wonder if this was a resonance of Ray energy, a kind of induced vibratory increase brought on through my close proximity to Professor Lovelock. Who knows? All I can say is that it made a lasting impression on me and taught me something vitally important about human beings and the effect we can have on each other. Most important was the sowing of a seed of recognition, which was to do with the power and transforming/stimulating potential of relationship, however brief.

The second occasion was during the Live Aid concert which I was watching on television — a truly global event. There was a particular point when Bob Geldof was singing: "I don't like Mondays ..." and he reached the line "...and the lesson today is how to die ...". Silence. I well remember the electric effect of that moment, aware myself that this moment mattered. I was choked, with tears in my eyes, hurting. Bob Geldof described in his book, *Is That It?*,[4] his need to will everyone to "please understand". It lasted only for a few seconds yet it stretched God knows where. We were all being offered an opportunity to open our hearts, to hurt, to care, to respond to need. Sadly, but perhaps inevitably, we so often have to be hurt into feeling *compassion*. Then comes the need for the wisdom and foresight to formulate responses that are truly helpful to the other

---

3.   World Goodwill is a service activity of the Lucis Trust that works to promote goodwill and service in the world, issuing a quarterly newsletter and a range of literature on a wide variety of topics.

4.   Bob Geldof, *Is That It?* (Penguin Books, London, 1986)

person, that are not simply a way of easing our personal discomfort. We all have many lessons to learn here.

It also shows the power in the moment. I believe we can create a focus within the collective mind and heart, which can impress the minds and hearts of individuals with ideas and feelings. Although it may seem that this kind of initiative has emerged out of increasing levels of communication and travel on a planetary level, the truth is that the idea is not new; it has been around for centuries. Many religious services have always been held on the same day and often at the same time. What is different is the idea of a global focus at the same moment in time.

I do not think we yet fully appreciate the power of thought and compassion when it is harnessed collectively and directed with love, intelligence and will. Perhaps we will discover more in the next century — I feel sure that we will. If, as I believe, energy does in some mysterious way follow thought (and probably feeling too), then we have within our minds and hearts the most powerful agent for change, transformation and growth. We simply have to realise it is there and then to train ourselves to use it, consciously, for the betterment of the human and planetary condition. However, it is not a substitute for practical action. The two must go hand in hand.

Becoming my own person

By the time I met Lynn I had already begun another cycle of experience in my life. I had participated in a week of group facilitation training with the Human Potential Resource Group at Surrey University which gave me a fresh insight into the nature of human relationships and human interaction and brought me into contact with the humanistic approach to counselling. It reached something deep inside me. You know how you sometimes touch, and are touched by, something that is extremely real and for you? It was one of those experiences, and I began to think of training in counselling.

Now, where do you start? Courses proliferate it seems almost by the second these days. I began with an evening class at a local Adult Education Centre. This gave me a basic understanding of some of the models of counselling, and allowed me to develop my relationship with this world a little more. I really was feeling my way at this time. Something was drawing me onwards, yet I knew it was not right to rush into anything. I needed to try to take a good deal of it in, so that I could make some informed choices. This is my style of approaching things: try to keep a balance between weighing up the information and listening to my heart.

These days I carry with me the motto: *The head directs, the heart connects*.

The next stage was a compressed training course with the Central School of Counselling and Therapy in Hackney, London. The skills element gave me a grounding in counselling interaction; the theory explored a whole range of approaches which included: psycho-dynamic; transactional analysis; gestalt and person- or client-centred.

I was drawn towards the Person-Centred Approach of Carl Rogers. During the course we had been shown a video of him demonstrating a counselling interview, and his humanity and genuine sensitivity towards the client made a deep impression on me. His way of working felt instinctively right. I certainly found it to be a truly human way of working and was beginning to reflect on my need for a counselling model that would enable me to connect with my spiritual ideas. I took the decision to look for a PCA course and enrolled with on a three-year diploma course[5] in Person-Centred Counselling and Psychotherapy.

Those three years brought me an amazing amount of insight and moved me on as a person in a way that I had not expected. My confidence and self-esteem certainly picked up, along with the ability to interact comfortably with others. My sensitivity to my own 'field of experiencing' grew. I left the Institute with something of a missionary zeal for bringing the PCA way of working into the world, well, at least into my world!

What I came away with most of all was a sense of my need to be able to be open in my communication and interaction with other people. I needed to be aware of what I was experiencing and be able to interpret it accurately in terms of its meaning. I also needed to be sensitive to the 'experiencing' of my clients and to create, through our relationship, a quality of interaction which would encourage them to take risks in their struggle to experience themselves in a more accurate way. Through this process they might gain fresh insight into their own nature and way of being.

As I became more and more absorbed in this approach, I found myself naturally wondering how the spiritual side of my world-view could be integrated into the PCA model and way of working. I was seeking a bridge between the strictly psychotherapeutic PCA and the possibility of becoming more than a person in the strictly human sense. Rogers wrote and spoke a great deal on the theme of "becoming a person". For me, we need to re-evaluate what we mean by a person: is it strictly limited to the flesh and blood experience of a physical form driven by chemical stimulus to reach as far as possible a state of full functionality? Or is it more? I believe it is more than this and that, within each of us, there exists a potential that I would term 'spiritual'.

5.   Run by The Institute for Person-Centre Learning, 220 Ashurst Drive, Barkingside, Essex, England IG6 1EW.

I sense that Rogers, as his life progressed, realised that the human organism is more, much more, than a biological entity. The passing over of his wife, Helen, had a deep effect on him and the following passage highlights his openness to larger possibilities.

> [my experiences] have made me much more open to the possibility of the continuation of the individual human spirit, something I had never before believed possible. These experiences have left me very much interested in all types of paranormal phenomena. They have quite changed my understanding of the process of dying. I now consider it possible that each of us is a continuing spiritual essence lasting over time, and occasionally incarnated in a human body.[6]

When I first read this passage I felt "yes!" being shouted from within my own Soul. This was the link I had sensed yet not previously found in Rogers' writings. It indicated for me the idea of a bridge between the human and the spiritual. It was a powerful moment for me, and it confirmed me in my quest. I knew then that I was on the right track.

Many have experienced a yearning for a deeper connection and for more meaningful relationships in which this inner, spiritual nature can be present. This union has been described using a variety of images, such as: the spark returning to the flame; the water droplet returning to the ocean. In the therapeutic relationship we can create an environment that touches this longing, creating a kind of re-membering of that which we know within us, yet which we have forgotten. Something very precious can be created, that reflects a quality of being and wholeness that transcends the normal round of human experience. Therapy is not merely a technique for overcoming blocks and problems but offers an opportunity for growth beyond becoming a person. It offers the opportunity of Soul-centred living.

Engaging with the spiritual aspect of my nature has, in truth, been the essence of my journey, carrying with it an urge to define a more 'Soul-centred psychology'. It would acknowledge our spirituality and the idea that we have, at the core of our psychological make-up, a Soul, a spiritual consciousness that transcends our normal awareness yet which we can access, experience and draw on. I see it as embodying qualities of love and compassion, existing in a state of wholeness that in some way transcends the individualistic nature. We are then part of an evolutionary process whose main thrust is the development and expansion of consciousness. I believe that life is about opening our hearts and minds to

6.   Carl Rogers, *A Way of Being* (Houghton Mifflin Co, Boston) pp. 91–2.

our Soul nature and allowing its essential qualities to find expression in our lives.

Moving on

I started to experience an increasing urge to reach out to people with the idea of the Seven Rays. It was in 1992, whilst I was seeking to publicise a workshop, that I met Lynn. This meeting was strange and yet, from the angle of connectedness, was not so strange.

A friend had sent me a piece of paper with names on it of people I might contact regarding publicity. The only person I did not know on the list was Lynn, so I rang her up late one Thursday evening. She was out and I had to leave a message on the answerphone. Lynn called back when she returned from her Circle Dance class and I arranged to go over and see her to hand over some flyers. I arrived on her doorstep the following Monday on my way home from work and was invited in.

We exchanged leaflets rather hastily because we each had appointments to keep. Hesitantly, knowing of the time constraints, Lynn asked, "would you like a cup of tea?". It seemed like a good excuse to stay a bit longer, so I replied, "Yes". Little did I know that my whole life was about to charge off on a completely new path! I still wonder what was really in the tea. After about 20 minutes we headed off in opposite directions.

The following evening I attended a talk at the Farnham New Age Group. Imagine my surprise as I sat down in the second row to find that the person next to me was ... Lynn! Ever get the feeling you are being pushed into something? Yet we were destined to go in different directions once more. The speaker wanted the chairs in a circle, and we headed off to opposite sides of the room! Strange to think that the first circle we shared required us to be opposite each other — the same positions we adopt now in our workshops.

We got back together again after the talk, would you believe over another cup of tea? The conversation flowed easily about the talk and the laughter exercises we had done. At the end of the evening we walked out into the car park, Lynn saying, "See you again sometime". "Sure," I replied.

Was it coincidence that we had met up again? We later discovered that we had both attended the same events at different times in our lives: festivals and other gatherings and yet there had been no contact between us. I had even been to a talk given by Lynn and she remembers me as being the one person in the room she did not speak to, yet somehow she knew our paths would cross again.

It seemed as though our relationship needed certain circumstances to be present in order to happen. We each had to have trodden our own individual paths to a particular point before we were in a certain sense ready to begin to journey together. Or maybe we needed to be shoved together!

I do find it fascinating to look back over life and to retrace the threads of connection that have brought us to the present. So often there are critical moments of decision, or so-called 'chance' meetings that have proved extremely significant. For many years I have had a sense that whatever I do there is an opportunity to carry some experience with me for future reference. The challenge is that we rarely know exactly what this something is at the time! Hence the need to be open to opportunities, and to accept experiences that maybe we do not like, but which, given eventual hindsight, are what we need. I believe strongly that we can either live our lives under the law of chance, or to some purpose. We can remain blind to the 'co-incidences' that occur and isolate ourselves from co-operating with what I would term 'Soul purpose', or we can accept that life is meaningful, that perhaps there are undercurrents moving us through life to bring us experience, and an opportunity to serve and to develop as a person. Somewhere I chose the latter during my teenage years and I have not regretted it.

Whilst life is a progression, moving through experiences which provide the opportunity for recognition and revelation, I am not sure that it is a linear process. I see it as a spiral path. Cyclically we face similar situations; each time, however, we are required to draw on some fresh revelation in order to grow out of the experience. So, whilst there is a sense of linear progression around and up the spiral, there are also connections from level to level. Wherever we are on the spiral of life, we are there for a purpose, for a lesson to be learned, a past experience to be seen and understood from a fresh vantage point. It is not that each successive phase is 'better' than a previous one. It simply leads us on towards ever greater revelation.

Spiritual teachings, if they are rooted in truth, are timeless and ever pertinent to the human condition. They also require to be worked at. In our instant world of 'soundbites' and 'quick-fix', we are drifting away from a culture that values concentration and sustained effort to achieve a goal. Spiritual growth is not an 'over the counter' remedy. It is a process of living, of exploring, of making mistakes (and hopefully learning from them), of being hurt and of being loved, of finding yourself and forgetting yourself, and finally of living in tune with the will and wisdom of the spiritual Self, the Soul.

Often we are blinded to the working out of this wisdom. We make choices, unaware of the significance they may have for a future time. About three weeks after our first meeting, I was at a loose end one evening, and felt I needed to go out, so I phoned Lynn again. We made a date and I went to check out a few places that I thought it would be nice to go to. I did not find what I was looking for, so I had to accept that the evening was going to be spontaneous. What I also did not know was that we were about to begin the journey together that has led to the workshops and writing this book.

Working Together

Richard

Our first evening out together was the night of the Leo full moon, and the weather was atrocious. Leo may be ruled by the sun but not that evening! The rain poured down as we headed out of Guildford. Waters may be symbolic of purification but you do not tend to think of this when you are getting drenched. We decided to just follow the bonnet of the car and see where we ended up — quite a wise decision because you could not actually see much beyond the bonnet. A few miles south of Guildford I said: "Have you got your passport?" A bewildered voice said, "No, why?". "Well, if we go on heading in this direction we'll reach the coast: we could go to France!" We decided to leave that for another time and turned off at the next set of traffic lights.

We finally arrived at a pub on the road between Hindhead and Farnham. My first memory of our arrival was the puddle. It and my foot converged in time and space. I cannot recall whether I had gallantly parked the car that way so that Lynn avoided the puddle, but I like to think so. Lynn, however, remembers the puddle on her side of the car, and the fact that she was wearing open-toed sandals!

The evening began in confusion. We ordered food and began to make to a table in the eating area. The waitress looked at me and enquired as to whether I was eating anything. Bemusement verging on panic must have crossed my face. Somehow we had managed to convey to her that Lynn wanted to eat but my preference had not made it to her pad. Was this symbolic of the future? Fortunately not, we both have a healthy interest in food and find ways of ensuring that our needs are met! With much relief I made my order and we set off to find a table.

It was not long before we were discussing Sacred Circle Dance and the Seven Rays. "I've been thinking," said Lynn, "about this idea of the Seven Rays. I'm sure I could put dances to each of those energies." She had been studying the leaflets I had left with her from our first meeting. "Great" I said, not knowing anything about the dances and wondering what I was letting myself in for.

I felt I could not contribute a great deal, but Lynn has a persistent streak when fired with enthusiasm. "Well, talk to me about the qualities of one of the Rays," she said. I talked of power, leadership, clarity, direction, determination — it was a wonder she stayed! With excitement in her voice she was soon describing a dance that demonstrated these aspects to a tee. I could sense that we were on to something and we were soon throwing ideas around in relation to all the Rays.

The discussion broadened out into life, the universe and how good the food was. The conversation was easy: we shared past experiences and discovered many common threads. I mentioned a festival in Brighton where I had had a stand some years back. "Was it at the Metropole?" asked Lynn. "Was there some Circle Dancing in the afternoon?" "Yes and yes". "I was there too," she announced, "and I was leading the dancing! Your stall was in the front left-hand corner wasn't it?" This was six or seven years previously: how had she remembered?

We both talked about the things that are really important to us: spiritual concepts, significant events, places we had visited. "If you had to make a list of special places to take someone, where would they be?", I asked. "Wimborne Minster, Avebury, the Lake District, and in Dorset the wishing well at Upwey and the petrified forest near Lulworth Cove. What about you?" My list was already in my head: "Avebury, Bamburgh Castle in Northumberland, the Black Mountains in South Wales, the White Horse at Uffington, Mam Tor in the Peak District, and Wastwater in the Lake District". Since then we have been to most of these 'special' places and shared our pleasure of them with each other.

Time passed. We did not notice how much and how quickly. The pub was closing and we were not exactly thrown out, but it was made clear that it was time to leave. I rather think that this was a good way to begin a new path and a curious setting for us to sow the seed of an idea. It seems funny now, looking back, that the seed got sown in a pub even though neither of us drink alcohol and I have now wound up as an alcohol counsellor.

When we got back to Lynn's flat she asked, "Would you like a cup of coffee?". "Yes, that would be nice, but I won't stay long." I noticed some familiar titles on Lynn's bookshelves: "I see you have some books by Yogi Ramacharaka". "Yes," came the reply from the kitchen. "And some by

David Spangler, even a few Sundial House publications," I called out. "One of them is on the Seven Rays," came the reply. Seeing such familiar titles made me feel quite at home! At three o'clock in the morning after further deep discussion and more cups of coffee, Lynn said "I've got to work tomorrow — or rather today!" So had I.

Much later, Lynn told me of her experience during the next day. "I felt as though a wind was rushing through my heart centre. It was as if I had opened up completely. I've never met anyone before that I could talk to so easily and openly about things that are really close to my heart." I, too, had been rocked by the intensity of it all, yet it felt really good.

Trust

It seemed from the start that there was a quality of trust present in our relationship, not simply trust of each other, but rather of a process and of the relationship that was forming. This is an important quality and one that we bring very much into our workshops. We have been reflecting on the nature of our relationship and how we function together both in, and out, of the workshop setting. We have tried to differentiate the two in our minds but realise that this is not possible. The relationship is what we bring into all that we do together, in all areas of our life. It is not a case of switching from 'domestic-mode' to 'workshop-mode'; we are who we are, together and as individuals, pretty much regardless of the setting.

Very early on we found that we could be completely open with each other about our lives, our interests, our search for meaning in life. It was a wonderful experience for us both to find this rapport, openness and mutual respect.

In the early days of our relationship I went through a learning process in how to speak from my own heart. I was the kind of person who could quote what other people had said on a whole range of topics. I remember a late-night discussion early on in which Lynn was expressing her thoughts and feelings. I actually lost track of what she was saying; what was making the impression was how she was speaking: "You really speak from your heart don't you?" I said. "It's so important for you to find the right words, your words." "Yes," she replied, "it has to come from me. I have to speak my own truth, not someone else's." Although it sometimes took time to find the right words, it was important for her to be able to do this.

I really respected this and it cast a contrasting light on me. I knew something had to change in me and this experience made the need more real. It became for me an intense need to find and to trust my own truth.

Other people's knowledge and insight are important, but they can only be a signpost.

Lynn challenged me a great deal over what I said, and why I said it. It has become increasingly important to speak from my own heart and to formulate my own ideas. Yes, I draw from other people's wisdom but I now realise that I have to discover and express my own knowledge and understanding.

Returning to the significance of trust, it is an incredibly important quality to develop and is something I have given a lot of reflective thought to. What do we trust? Who do we trust? Do we trust *in* something? How do our expectations fit in with trust? I am not so sure that we trust *in* anything, rather it is about trusting the process of life. I believe there is a purpose in life and that we can trust that it is taking us where we need to be. We may not always like where it takes us, but I think that, if we can keep in step with it, we will discover opportunities to grow and to serve.

There was an episode in the first series of 'Star Trek' where McCoy had gone back into the past and had carried out an act that had changed the future. Kirk and Spock had to go back to roughly that same time and prevent whatever McCoy had done from happening. Kirk's comment was something to the effect that time flowed and would take you where you were meant to be. The implication was that, because McCoy and later he and Spock, were stepping into a similar flow of time then their paths would cross. I think we do flow along a time-continuum. What that means exactly, I do not know! But it can be trusted to somehow take us where we need to be, along with others whom we need to meet and interact with.

In many ways I find myself moving more towards an attitude of acceptance with regard to trust. This is not, however, a negative or passive condition. I accept the process but that does not mean I accept the human condition or that I am not motivated to want to do something to help people. I have observed a passive attitude around that seems to accept things as they are and that all will be well, as if we can remain as mere spectators. Maybe it will all be well, but we have to be more than spectators; surely we have to be participants within the human drama, strenuously playing our part to encourage values of selflessness and harmlessness, responsibility and compassion. We have to participate. Spirituality is about finding and living your grasp of Truth. It requires energy, direction and purpose — the fire of love.

First steps

"Would it be alright if I came to your Tuesday class?" I asked Lynn tentatively one day, remembering my platform boots! "That would be great," she replied. So when people ask us how we choose the dances for our workshops we reply that it is a matter of experiencing them. Initially, I joined Lynn's groups and fed back to her which dances seemed to capture something of the different qualities of Ray energy. At the same time, we were talking and discussing the Rays, so Lynn's knowledge was developing too. After each dance class we would go through the list and work out whether they really fitted with particular energies.

"What was that one where we did all the weaving into the centre?"

"Do you mean Lamiita?"

"Probably, how does it go?"

Lynn demonstrates round the furniture!

"Yes, that's the one. It feels very third Ray to me. What about the gentle one with the hesitant step towards the centre that we began with?"

"You mean Arouna Pleven, the one danced in an open circle?"

"That's it. That feels like a second Ray dance, it really left me with a sense of gentle persistence and close connection with the group."

So that is how it evolved. After direct experience of the dance we discussed which of them fitted our pattern. Sometimes it was certain movements, or direction of movement, sometimes it was the speed or slowness of the music, or the rhythm and the harmony. Often it was the feelings that the dance left us with. It was an exciting time for us both.

I remember when I first saw Lynn dance. "You're not watching what I'm doing," she suddenly said, somewhat accusingly. "Hmm, sorry," I replied. "It's just that you change when you dance, it's as if your whole body smiles." It had made such an impression on me. Later Lynn told me that I had a rather glazed look in my eyes. I had lost track of the steps and what we were doing. I guess I had had my first taste of the transforming power of dance, in Lynn's living room amongst the chairs, settee and coffee table!

In partnership

The months passed and early the following year we were in Guildford one Saturday morning and found ourselves looking at an estate agent's window display. "That looks rather nice," I said looking at a three-bedroom detached house in Woking. Lynn came across and peered over my shoulder. "Mm" she said, "It's not expensive either." I heard myself saying "Let's go and get the details". It was when we were on our way to view the property that Lynn said "You do realise that there are implications to this, don't you? Are you suggesting that we should live together?" "Well it would be nice, wouldn't it?" I said, and regretted it immediately when Lynn said in a rather hurt voice, "I think I'd like it to be more than *nice*!"

There was something quite unemotional about it all, as though it simply made sense and was where life was taking us. It somehow seemed the reasonable thing to do in the light of how our relationship had developed. We did not end up buying the house we looked at that day, but we now knew that it was only a matter of time before we bought a home together. We had somehow decided to share our lives without discussing it first. It was a decision that grew out of a love that, whilst full of feeling, was not of the 'fizzy' kind. Beware of bubbly love, it has a horrible tendency of going flat on you.

Trust and acceptance played a large part in our search for a home. After a number of months we found one that seemed to fit our requirements, made an offer and waited. Our offer was not accepted, yet within a couple of weeks we found somewhere else one evening much more suited to our needs. In fact, it was a house we looked at simply because it was close to another one that we planned to see that evening.

We moved into this house together three days after our first workshop dancing the Seven Rays. Looking back now we think that, whilst it was not what we had planned, maybe the concern about the move served to keep us from being anxious about the workshop, and our worries about the workshop kept us from being too apprehensive about the move! Anyway, both went off well and in Part 4 we describe how *Dancing the Sevenfold Energies of Life* has taken form and evolved.

This sequence of events showed us how the life-process sometimes blocks us from a particular direction in a clear and unequivocal manner. We may have our plans but the form that they take may need to change. We have to be prepared to adapt and adjust whilst holding our sense of direction clearly in our minds and hearts. We may know where we are going, but the journey may take an unexpected route. We may even end up somewhere else, but we need a sense of direction.

Group work

Our attitude towards the workshops comes back to trust and the quality of relationship that we have built together. We trust the participants implicitly as persons in their own right, and the process of growth and learning that they are experiencing, which has drawn them to share in a day or weekend with us. We also trust each other, allowing space to express ourselves in the workshop and to compensate for each other. It is not that we are trying to impose a certain way of being on the group setting, we simply seek to be ourselves as persons in relationship. I wonder sometimes whether it all boils down not so much to striving to *do* as to *be*, a way of being that is present and participative and from which doing can proceed — letting our 'human doing' proceed out of our 'human being'.

I believe that group facilitators hold more power than they sometimes realise. It seems that what they bring into the group gets mirrored and magnified into the group experience. I have seen this occur too many times to dismiss it lightly. Not just in therapeutic groups. Managers also affect their teams in this way.

In our work we seek to be ourselves and not to play games with people. We take what we do seriously but try not to take ourselves too seriously. Humour plays an important part in this. I see a sense of humour as being a crucial feature of the human person. We use it a lot in the workshops — not in a planned way, generally it happens spontaneously. It can help promote learning because it helps people to open up in themselves. A healthy sense of humour that is not of the 'laughing at', but of the 'laughing with', kind is expressive of a sense of proportion. We do get life out of proportion sometimes. We do inflate our own importance and our own issues. We do need to learn to 'sit light in the saddle'.

We are also not aiming to give anyone anything. It is not a lecture format that we are seeking to create, rather a space for people to experience something of themselves that is new and refreshing. We do not know what people will take away from a day or a weekend with us. I well remember one occasion when we had put a lot of work into researching the theme and, when we invited participants to share their expectations and hopes for the day, we heard:

"I want a day off."
"I just want to have fun."
"I facilitate workshops all the time and I need some space with someone else doing the work!"
"I need some time just for me"
"I'm just glad to be here and be open to whatever happens."
"I want to dance and enjoy myself."

It went on like that all round the circle. Nobody seemed particularly interested in the technicalities of the subject: they all wanted time to be themselves. It seemed everyone had come along because they needed a day off from their own work (they were mostly people who facilitated groups of their own): they just wanted to enjoy themselves!

Dance as a mirror

An image we have is of the dance being like a mirror. When you stand in front of a mirror, what do you see? You see a reflection of yourself. In the same way, when we bring ourselves into the dance we see ourselves reflected in it. Yet it is more than a reflection: it is a direct experience of who we are and how we function. It is intensely personal: our own recognition of our own individual qualities. Nobody else has the same experience, yet we can share it with the rest of the group. However, the mirror reflects a two-dimensional image and allows us to see only what is on the surface. The dance enables us to go deeper, to touch and be touched by the invisible processes that shape our character and sense of self. In a strange and mysterious way it is like stepping into the mirror, allowing us to form a close and more intimate relationship with ourselves.

Added to this, there are occasions when people in the group notice mannerisms reflected in the movements of another participant of which he/she is unaware, yet which have a significance for that individual's way of being. So we have the dual aspect of looking at and stepping into our own mirror, and of others observing us.

The wonderful thing about group work is that people can take away from the experience more than they came with. This is important. Also, because of the number of people in the group, each with insight and experience to share, participants are given an opportunity to glean a great deal from a variety of perspectives.

We see ourselves throwing out seeds of ideas to people. Someone once described it: "I see you as throwing out threads of light for people to catch." I think this is probably quite accurate. We do not know what will be conveyed in a workshop that will prove to have particular meaning for each individual. We seek to be open to the moment in such a way that deeper communication can occur, which can be either inter- or intra-personal (or both). Indeed, it can stretch into the transpersonal too, bringing a whole new dimension and dynamic into the group relationship. The more the facilitator can be true to themselves, open to the experience around and within them, and be accurate in their interpretation of their experience, the greater the possibility that a growth-enhancing process will take place in the group. It is then that the adventure really begins.

Part 2

Sacred Circle Dance

by Lynn

*Sacred Circle Dance has an amazing ability
to make me feel whole, to give me strength
and the courage to cope with the stresses of life*

Origins of Sacred Circle Dance

The original collection of Sacred Circle Dances was made by Bernhard Wosien, who was a German dance professor. He travelled to Greece and former Yugoslavia and learned their folk dances. Realising that he had something very important he searched for a suitable place to take them where they would be appreciated. He knew they created a very special atmosphere and a feeling of group cohesion and harmony which he thought was unique in our busy everyday lives.

Many of the dances celebrate significant events in the life of a community: weddings, births, deaths both of people and animals, the agricultural cycle and the connection of humanity with Nature and the Divine. In the countries of origin many of them may be considered to be dances of 'rites of passage'.

Findhorn

Eventually, in 1976, he was invited to share them with the Findhorn spiritual community in Scotland, where they became a fact of life. This community was started in the 1960s by Peter and Eileen Caddy and Dorothy Maclean. After an extraordinary set of circumstances they found themselves in a small caravan on a site in sand dunes by Findhorn Bay on the North-East coast. In this desolate place they became famous for growing their own vegetables in soil that 'should not' have grown anything. And they were no ordinary vegetables: 40 pound cabbages were the norm!

These achievements, as a result of meditation and acceptance that a higher power was in charge of the Plan, made the three adults and three children famous. People started to flock there to enrich their spiritual life and to find a meaning that had escaped them before. It was not long before a community of like-minded people sprang up. In this context, Bernhard Wosien took his collection of dances to Findhorn which he described as a "fertile ground" where "they would flourish". Today the community is in the hundreds, ecological houses have been built and a universal hall — and they still dance!

Bernhard had called his dances *Heilige Tanze*. In German, *heilige* means holy or sacred; it also has connotations of healing and wholeness. The English translation of 'sacred' is inadequate and we have no single word to cover the multiplicity of meaning of the German word. Bernhard wrote of these dances:

"One has to dance them and be totally present to discover their meaning and healing power. Only then does their religious origin reveal itself — the way to Oneness, from separation to community to vibrant togetherness."[7]

This is the power of the dance — to bring people together, to create harmony among a group of near strangers. Many aspects of modern life seem to me to separate us from each other: these dances encourage a renewed sense of community.

Then the dances spread

A community is inevitably a changing entity and people left Findhorn to start new lives elsewhere, inspired by the philosophy and spirituality they had encountered. They took with them the Sacred Circle Dances. One of the first teachers, David Roberts, luckily for me, lived in the South East of England. He started many groups which grew and flourished. The one in Washington, West Sussex is still alive today after various changes of teacher.

Gradually the word was spreading and the wonderful feeling generated by this type of movement together was a necessary part of life for an increasing number of people. To those who have not come across Sacred Circle Dance this may sound a strange way of describing it. I hear you say "it sounds like an addiction". Well, maybe it is! But surely it is a very healthy one that is not going to do any damage to anyone and will bring pleasure and joy to many.

Sacred Circle Dance today

We dance in a circle, usually holding hands, so you do not need a partner, and the intention is for everyone to do the same steps. This sounds so simple, and it is! Just making this connection can be the beginning of a journey of self-discovery. The effect is enhanced by everyone moving together to beautiful music, making a kaleidoscope of patterns on the floor.

Over the years hundreds more dances have been added. There was a time when every teacher knew the same dances, but that is no longer true. It depends where you have been and who you have danced with. Some of the dances are traditional, from countries such as Greece, Romania, Bulgaria, Israel, France, Russia — in fact anywhere that they dance in circles!

---

7.   Bernhard Wosien, "*A life lived for dance*".

There is also a huge number of newly choreographed dances. Some-one may hear a piece of music that really inspires them and they will put steps to it: another dance is born.

Dance as an immediate experience

Sacred Circle Dances come in many guises from the gentle to the asser-tive, from the slow to the fast, and from the simple to the complex. They are a wonderful means of expression: for instance, we can experience in a very immediate way the vitality of spring in a fast dance such as Le Printemps from France; we feel for the young girl entering marriage when we do the thoughtful bride's dance, Odano Oro from Macedonia; we feel deep tenderness, love and gratitude in the Israeli dance, Ahawat Hadassa, to a beloved niece; and we can even acknowledge our own feelings of aggression when we dance like a warrior in Arap from former Yugoslavia (and this is surely a safe way to express this type of emotion).

The recent choreographies add another dimension to the experience. We can fly like the White Bird to atmospheric music on pan pipes from South America; we know what it is like to open and close like a flower with the sun in the Dandelion Dance; and we celebrate the joy of life in Hallelujah Elohim.

If you have never Circle Danced, do try it. It is a wonderful experi-ence, but be prepared to get hooked!

Sacred Space —Walls do have Ears

Of course the whole of the planet is sacred space but we rarely treat it as such. People designate special sites as being sacred, because they 'feel' good. Yet what is that feeling and how was it created in the first place? Is it a natural phenomenon to do with the location, either in terms of geo-graphical position or height (these sites often seem to be on the tops of hills, but then being above the surrounding countryside, wherever you are, is an exhilarating experience)? In this chapter I offer a means of cre-ating sacred space based on my experience with Sacred Circle Dance.

Energy of the dance

Holding hands in a circle and moving in unison to music creates a sense of community, of belonging, that is very healing. Many people do not experience this harmony in any other part of their life.

We usually dance round a candle in the centre of the circle. One of the most moving times for me is when we turn out the electric light for the last dance of the evening. The central candle gives us quite sufficient light to dance by and it is soft and gentle in comparison with the harsh electric bulbs.

As we dance by candlelight, there is a second line of dancers that copy exactly what we do, but in a circle beyond ours that moves round the walls and over the ceiling. These dancers are our own shadows. They have a very protective feeling about them. Our shadows become our guardian angels — this gives a new meaning to the 'shadow' aspect of ourselves, seen in the light of the candle. They shield us from harm and move with us in perfect harmony. They fade when the artificial light comes on again but their energy is left in the walls.

Walls do have ears ...

Since starting to teach Sacred Circle Dance in 1983, an interesting phenomenon has set me thinking. In the early days it was often difficult to teach even the simplest of dances: people stumbled and struggled and generally looked as though they had two left feet (there were exceptions, of course!). This has gradually changed over the years and now I teach complicated dances to near beginners and they pick them up remarkably quickly. What has happened? Obviously I have become more experienced as a teacher but I feel there is more to it than that.

Does the hundredth monkey syndrome[8] also apply to learning dances? Certainly the number of dancers has increased dramatically. In 1983 there were only a handful of teachers with maybe a couple of regular groups each. Now there are groups all over the country and the list of teachers extends to three and a half pages of small print in the Network Journal *Grapevine*. So the hundredth monkey syndrome must play a part in the ease with which people learn the steps.

---

8. Some years ago scientists were investigating the behaviour patterns of monkeys on a series of islands. They fed them sweet potatoes and one of the female monkeys suddenly went to the sea and washed her potatoes. Soon the other monkeys on that island followed suit. This in itself was not surprising, but it was then discovered that when the hundredth monkey started to clean potatoes the troupe on the next island also started to wash theirs. A pattern of behaviour had been established in a remote community seemingly by virtue of the number of monkeys adopting that pattern elsewhere. We have also seen this occur among the tit population with regard to pecking the tops out of milk bottles to access the cream.

There also seems to be a greater consciousness of the need for community. It is an aspect of our lives that has been neglected for a long time; we have all led our separate lives without much consideration for others or for group activities. Now people are reaching out for each other and are enthusiastic about entering into a communal spirit — the silent giving and receiving of the circle is a powerful influence on their lives.

However, I have another theory for your contemplation: that the room in which I dance plays a large part in all this. I have noticed that when I use a new hall I experience greater difficulty in conveying the steps. Do the walls have memory? Do the bricks hold energy from previous dance sessions? It is an awe-inspiring thought but that appears to be exactly what is happening. So maybe the walls *do* have ears.

We have probably all experienced walking into a room and suddenly being overcome with a sense of foreboding or, on the opposite end of the scale, a lightness and joyfulness. Most people will buy a house only if it 'feels good'. This is no mere superstition surely. Walking into a cathedral or a department store are different experiences. Why? Places of prayer and meditation feel peaceful; they take us away from the hustle and bustle of everyday life. The big shopping precinct takes us right back into the midst of it.

Do we pick up on the events that have occurred within those four walls previously? The energy of earlier occurrences may reside in the fabric of the building. So is it too far-fetched to suppose that the energy of our dancing is held in the walls of the rooms we use? I do not think so.

Powerful emotions

After all, as we have seen, the dances can represent powerful aspects of people's lives. Sacred Circle Dance can bring us back in touch with these turning points of life. The energy generated when dancing out such momentous events in a circle and all holding hands is very powerful: it can elate the dancers, it can reduce people to tears, it helps others to contact their hidden emotions. It can empower and inspire them to take new and positive directions in their own path that had not been considered previously — I know, it has happened to me!

So is it surprising that the room retains some of that energy when we depart? If it holds the emotion of these experiences surely it can also store the energy of the steps we dance. The patterns of the sequences are then available to tap into when that group (or another) meets again. The room becomes a dancer amongst us. The magic is not only in the air.

More than that, the walls surround us when we dance: they are protecting us and give of their energy to us from an outer 'circle'. If you have ever sat at the centre of a circle of people holding hands you will know what a powerful experience it can be. The feeling of comfort, protection and upliftment is very strong. I believe this happens to us all in a room that is used consistently for this type of group experience.

The most commonly expressed effect of the dances seems to be a sense of healing. The very fact of being in a circle and holding hands can produce this feeling: the movement to music enhances it. If my theory is correct, this healing energy is stored in the walls of the room. I am suggesting that the energy the dances create is not only available to dancers to make it easier for them to learn sequences; it is there for all to experience who enter the room. It is an awesome thought and gives us dancers a great sense of responsibility, yet it is happening without our necessarily realising it!

Sacred Circle Dance seems to be helping to start a new movement towards community, towards co-operation. In the dances we have to work together to create the atmosphere and the effect. Yet it is possible to dance without this sense of companionship and collaboration. When we recognise this we see our responsibility clearly. If the walls have a 'memory' they will not only remember the 'good', but the 'bad and the ugly' as well. Our separative and selfish feelings can be magnified in the walls in just the same way as those of harmony and unity. People revisiting Auschwitz experience the terrible atmosphere that still exists. The energy of the evil perpetrated there still remains. This is an extreme example, but it illustrates my point.

This implies that we need to be totally aware wherever we are and whatever we do. The walls at least will be listening and remembering.

Sacred sites and ley lines

This then is one way to create sacred space. To be conscious that whatever we do is recorded in the building or the ground on which we walk, and be mindful that we each leave our mark, our energy, wherever we go. It leaves us with an awesome responsibility but then that is true just because we are here on Earth, living with awareness and following a spiritual path. The energy of Sacred Circle Dance can be used to enhance this effect.

If we are creating a sacred space when we dance — a space in which the healing energy of the dance is retained and is accessible by any who enter — it makes me wonder whether the sacred sites of the ancient Celts may have been created by 'dancing energy into them'. We know that dance was an important part of 'religious' ceremony in times past. It is said, for instance, that the stone circles were danced around and within.

This leads me to ponder which came first — the sacred sites or the ley lines connecting them? It may be that the ancient sacred sites were created in this way by recognising the energy and the effect of the dance. It would be automatic then for the energy to flow between sites as it does in an electric circuit.

We can picture this as the dance inducing an energy flow much like acupuncture does. By adjusting the flow of energy in a particular meridian of the body the acupuncturist helps the overall functioning of that person. Is it the dance — the movement, the vibration/rhythm of the contact with the Earth — or the relationship created between the dancers that acts as the acupuncture/acupressure? Maybe it is both because in truth they cannot be separated. One cannot exist without the other.

Personal experience

I led some Sacred Circle Dancing at a Fountain International[9] conference some years ago. We were outside dancing in a courtyard with two ley lines crossing in the centre of the circle. There were several dowsers there and they were measuring the energy levels. These rose first of all when we joined hands: when we started dancing they were magnified many times.

Perhaps more surprisingly, the flow of the energy in the ley lines was also affected. At the beginning the flow was straight in both lines. By the end of the dancing the dowsers were reporting that the energy was flowing to the centre in the same way as before but was redirected to one outlet only — in fact towards a little chapel which was on one of the original lines. So there is some evidence that the energy flow is influenced when we dance in this way.

Conclusion

It is fascinating to speculate like this, yet for me it really is not important to know the 'answers' in a scientific way. Change is definitely occurring and Sacred Circle Dance has become an element in that change for many

---

9.   Fountain International is an organisation founded by Colin Bloy many years ago to focus light and love to the planet. It originated in Brighton with the idea of concentrating on the fountain there as a focal point for the town, to bring healing and health to the neighbourhood. The effect was found to be astonishing and other groups sprang up in England and around the world. Reports of the results include reduction of crime, and a happier and healthier population. This just by focusing positive energy to an agreed focal point.

people. We are creating a sense of belonging through dance, in the atmosphere of human 'being'. This surely is creating sacred space.

Having acknowledged the power of these dances, maybe the challenge is to apply it consciously to lifting the atmosphere in demanding environments such as schools, businesses, prisons and community centres.

Sacred Dance and Spirituality

Dance in many forms has been used over the ages as an expression of the deepest aspects of life, of the dancer's relationship with the Earth, the animal and vegetable kingdoms, and, perhaps most importantly, the connection with the Divine. In tribal societies, dance is a natural means of communication: it expresses joy, sadness, love and hate; it instils power in an invading tribe; it pleads with the gods to provide food, rain, sun; it celebrates the 'rites of passage' — birth, puberty, initiation, marriage, death.

What has happened to dance in our modern society? Over the last few decades we have seen the gradual separation of the people dancing. We have a heritage of British Folk Dance, yet few young people know any of these dances (except possibly in Scotland which seems to have retained its dancing tradition). There is occasionally a barn dance or ceilidh, which provides the opportunity for community dancing, yet it often disintegrates into a muddle of uncoordinated movement.

Ballroom dancing is a delightful means of communication, the gliding steps and the closeness of the partners giving a feeling of flowing with life. Yet how often do people dance like that these days? Even a 'dinner dance' turns out to be bopping to a disco. There is no band and the old familiar dance rhythms are not apparent to me. The dancing is done individually with little or no contact either physically or mentally with other people.

I think the increasing popularity of Sacred Circle Dance in this country demonstrates a need for people to recapture some of the spirituality of dance. We are in a circle holding hands; the intention is for everyone to do the same steps. This surely is an expression of spirituality, acknowledging our inter-connectedness with each other and the Divine.

Experiencing connection

There is no separation in the circle. All participants are equal. Well I think it is more accurate to say that we are the same but different! The circle depends on the contribution of each of its members: each is important and each is necessary to the working of the whole. So, while there is connection, there is also individual movement and personal expression of the steps. The atmosphere of the dance is experienced differently by everyone. Looking round a dancing circle this is very apparent. There are the people who like to get the dance 'right' and copy the teacher to the very best of their ability. Then there are those who, come what may, are going to interpret the dance in their own unique style. It may be nothing like the original dance but that is immaterial to them. So there is unanimity but not uniformity; we each express the same dance in our own unique way.

Similarly the goal in life is not uniformity but unanimity. In any group, to achieve a common spirit with one another and a sense of unity is a powerful experience. We have all touched the same place within us, a common place, and from each of us that essence flows through the coloured glass of our own personality. This is the dance of life. In Sacred Dance we experience this unanimity and know that it is possible in a more global sense. We all move towards the centre of the circle, symbolising the spiritual goal; we each approach differently but the intention is the same.

The circle gains a momentum of its own. It becomes a single entity and the whole is greater than the sum of the parts. The essence of Sacred Dance is felt when as individuals we can allow ourselves 'to be danced'. The head no longer tries to remember the steps or the pattern; the memory is in the body and the dance becomes a meditation. We all move together in harmony and the simplest dance becomes a powerful expression of that greater unity. There seems to be a 'muscle memory' that allows us to dance in this way, free of the restrictions of the mind and its constant analysis. The dance takes us over, the muscles remember what they did to this tune before and repeat the movements. We are then free to experience the essence or quality of the dance that lies behind the outer form of movement.

In the dance we are united, yet we retain our uniqueness, we are each a part of the integrated whole while maintaining our individual integrity. This is a direct expression in form of the nature of our association with each other on this planet and with Divinity. We are like the dancers in a circle — moving together for the common good, yet each playing our own part. We all have a role to play, and the whole is not complete unless we do it to the best of our ability. A circle that is broken is disjointed and does not flow. We have to co-operate with each other to create an environment in which to experience the depth and meaning of the movement. That is not easy. We make mistakes: yet that is alright too! In time, we find our feet and our place within the greater whole.

Whilst we all attempt to dance the same steps, it is the flow of the movement which is so vital. It is advisable for practical reasons to all move in the same direction; on a spiritual level this is translated into the intention to work towards the same goal — that of creating an atmosphere of peace and harmony, joy and vitality. It is as if the dance becomes a microcosm of our journey in life: if we flow with each other, a feeling of well-being and connection is generated; if we resist or fight against our neighbour, disharmony and tension are in evidence.

Facing in and out

A fascinating aspect of the circle is the difference we experience when we are facing towards the centre of the circle and when we face outwards. In some dances we turn round and repeat a sequence of steps that we have just done facing inwards. Invariably it is more difficult for people to learn the steps when they have their backs to the candle, yet they are the same movements, we are just facing a different direction.

Perhaps when we all face the centre we are concentrating the energy towards that centre and are able to tap into it in some way. We can watch the movements of the other people in the circle. When we face out all our energy is dissipated out to the rest of the world and some of the focus is lost: we no longer have the comfort and security of being a member of a group.

This gives us some insight into our everyday lives. We need the strength and support of our group of friends; we need that focus. When we go out into the world alone we may stumble and take wrong turnings. Again we come back to the idea of individuals within a unity. On our own we can lose the steps of life: when we turn to face the group again our energy and direction become clearer.

At another level it is about allowing ourselves time and space to reconnect with our centre and the source of our energy and direction. Then we are again strong enough spiritually to take the next step out into the world. I see the candle in the centre representing my own inner light in my own centre. Sometimes when I am 'facing out into the world' I seem to lose sight of that light and focus. I need to make a conscious effort to turn back to it, to reinforce my spirituality and be able to use it wisely and well.

We find time and again that Sacred Circle Dance is a microcosm of the macrocosm of our lives. It teaches us about ourselves, our aspirations, our abilities and our blocks. We can carry the lessons we thus learn into the rest of our lives and grow as a result of our experience.

"You must be the change you wish to see in the world" said Gandhi. This is surely what living spiritually is all about.

Dance and religion

Dance has been an integral part of religious life in many countries and many faiths. Yet in Britain today it seems to be largely frowned upon by the Church. David danced for joy round the Ark, apparently in a 'circle dance' denoting the motion of the planets round the sun. In the Gnostic Gospels there is the image of Jesus asking his disciples to dance round him in a circle prior to his betrayal, to give him the energy to go through with what was being asked of him. So why is dance so often thought now to be sacrilege in Church?

This reminds me of the story of a Sacred Dance teacher leading a large group of people in a few dances many years ago. Some of those attending did not want to participate: of the onlookers one was heard to say to her neighbour, "I don't know what's sacred about this — they look as though they're enjoying themselves to me"! It seems as if religion, spirituality and sacredness have become, for some, synonymous with dullness, seriousness and heaviness. Yet surely there are many things to celebrate and life was not meant to be all hard toil and no joy. "Life is for living" as the saying goes and what better way to express that life than in dance.

Of course there has to be a balance between work and play. This, too, is expressed in Sacred Dance. There has to be a balance between mastering the steps to the best of our ability, and the sheer joy of moving together in rhythm. When the pattern becomes a part of us and there is no more toil in learning, then we can experience the full essence of the dance. The body seems to almost burst with the exhilaration of the movement, and the dance takes us to a different level of being.

Moving mandala

We come to the circle individually. We stand on our own in a circle. The connection with the Divine can be visualised as running from our head centre through our heart centre and down to our feet. We are each a link between 'heaven' and 'earth'. Our individual threads meet above the centre of the circle and the spiritual unity of the group is automatic.

Then we reach out to our neighbours on either side and join hands, thus making the connection one with the other and completing the circle. The thread this time runs from one hand to the other through the heart centre. The common point is found in the heart and we have a vertical and a horizontal line running through each of us forming an equal-armed cross, which represents the relationship of four equal things — the seasons, the poles, the kingdoms...

In this way we create the powerful ancient symbol of the circle and the cross, which seems to represent so many different aspects of life, including the manifest within the unmanifest, and polarity within the wholeness. The fascinating thing is that there is another, or rather many other, such patterns. We make connections all round the circle from our own heart centre to that on the opposite side. There is a myriad of circle and cross symbols all round the group, overlapping and interweaving. The vertical cross and horizontal circle pass through the individual heart centre. The horizontal cross and circle have a common point at the centre of the circle — the heart centre of the group.

We then dance and become a moving mandala. We trace intricate and beautiful patterns on the floor: I have often thought it would be wonderful to have coloured chalk on our feet so that we could see the details of the designs. Yet it is not only the patterns we make on the floor that are significant; it is the totality of the movements combining to make a three-dimensional living creation. Mandalas have been used in many cultures to focus the energy and create a deeper relationship with the Divine. The candle provides a lovely centrepiece so that the circle stays in the same place in the room. Yet also a candle is used in a particular form of meditation as a focus. So here we are bringing together different ways of allowing spirit into our lives. The unity of movement, the candle at the centre, and the patterns we create bring us into a different relationship with each other and the spiritual part of our nature.

Energy of the circle

Another remarkable effect is the energy that dancing generates. Some people cannot imagine being able to summon up enough stamina to dance most of the day, and yet they not only can do it but feel energised rather than depleted at the end of it. In the circle we hold hands with one palm up and the other down. This allows the energy to flow right round the circle from person to person. We are continually exchanging energy and there have been many instances of the healing effect of this. There is no intentional healing taking place: it is a natural consequence of the joining of hands and the resulting flow of energy.

It seems this can happen in the most unlikely circumstances: I have watched ME (chronic fatigue syndrome) sufferers apparently changing as they enter into the joy and vitality of the dance. I have witnessed similar transformations in people with other symptoms of illness.

From my experience I would say there are various forms of tiredness. There is the exhaustion that we may feel at the end of a day of work: this can certainly be overcome by a couple of hours of Sacred Circle Dance. People talk of coming to an evening class when they are absolutely exhausted or have a headache – they could hardly drag themselves out of the chair. Yet after a few dances they have revived and found a new lease of life. The difficult thing in these circumstances seems to be getting the energy to leave the house in the first place!

It seems to be a paradox that movement, sometimes extremely energetic, and often a little taxing mentally, should bring renewed energy, yet that is what we experience in the circle. Afterwards there may be a tiredness but it is of a different nature: now it is accompanied by a sense of elation. It is hard to describe but I know the difference in feeling.

Another effect is that we create an energy at the centre, when we move in unison. Animals seem to be particularly sensitive to this. On many occasions I have been in a dancing circle when a cat or a dog has come from who knows where and sat in the centre. One of these times the dog was licking his paw when we arrived to dance in the open air. He appeared to be quite distressed. We started dancing and the dog got up, limped right into the centre and laid down. He no longer licked himself; he looked as though he was bathing in the healing effect of his central position. Just as suddenly he got up and walked away apparently no longer bothered by his paw. It was truly astonishing and yet felt quite natural.

When the dancing stops

The moment immediately after a dance is most important, because in that time we can really know what that dance meant to us personally. We do not clap, however much we may have enjoyed it. Random clapping dissipates the energy immediately and the essence of the dance is lost in an instant. Sometimes we use a native American Indian form of appreciation which is to wave our hands in the air above our heads. Thus we acknowledge our enjoyment without destroying the energy we have created. However, more often we simply hold the circle in stillness, reflecting quietly on our individual experience. There is a sense in which the moment after the movement captures the essence of the dance itself. The silence then is extremely poignant and much can be learnt in that time.

At the end of a session of Sacred Dance we hold the quiet and consciously direct the light of the candle, to bring healing and comfort to a particular part of the world or to somebody we know who is in need of positive thought. Blowing out the candle symbolises sending the energy from the centre out to the world. This is an important and beautiful moment: on a global level it helps to bring light down to Earth; on a personal level it reconnects us with our own environment after the uplifting experience of the dance. We are 'earthed' again.

People have remarked on the efficacy of this simple ritual. Sometimes we blow out the candle to one of our number who has not been able to come because of illness. On many occasions they report back that: "at half past nine I woke up and felt a surge of energy running through me"; or "I suddenly felt this amazing sense of warmth and joy, and when I looked at the clock it was just after 9.30". It is real, powerful and healing.

There is no doubt in my mind that Sacred Circle Dance is a spiritual expression, yet I rarely talk in these terms when I am teaching because it is important that everyone finds what the dance is for them.

Symbolism in the Circle

The circle has been known to be a powerful symbol since very early times. What is it that makes it so special? Perhaps for many ancient people it represented the shape of the most important part of their lives — the Sun, the source of heat and light, revered as the source of life itself. Hence the Sun was worshipped. The Moon was also seen to be circular and that was the compensating force of gentleness and beauty. We now know that the Earth is nearly spherical too. So the circle imitated these essential aspects of life.

We know that the Sun and the Earth have vast storehouses of energy deep within them. Sometimes this bursts forth, unable to be contained any longer, and we have sun spots and volcanoes. In a sense the humble circle mirrors this as well, for when we meet in circular form we concentrate energy at the centre. As we stand there the energy grows because we are all directing our heart centre towards the middle of the circle.

Paradoxical circle

The circle is an interesting figure from the mathematical point of view. If we measure its radius and attempt to calculate the circumference or area, we can only come to a close approximation, based on the elusive constant pi, which is not resolvable. Inversely, if we measure the circumference, we can only calculate the radius to the nearest so many decimal places. This makes the circle a magical construct which defies logical thought.

The circle has no beginning and no end: it represents infinity and becomes a symbol for the divine, the spiritual and the intangible. Yet at the same time it is all-encompassing. The feeling of inclusiveness when in a circle is remarkable: the difference between being in a group sitting in a circle and one sitting in straight lines is incredible. In a circle, we can all see each other; we experience some of what they experience; everyone is in the 'front row'. We are connected. We are strong together.

Yet there is another aspect to this. What of the person who walks into a room and sees a circle already formed? Is it easy to join that circle? It can often be very intimidating and there can be a feeling of exclusion. It is important when we are dancing to be aware of the presence of the newcomer; welcome them; bring them into the group; encourage them to feel secure. The group's strength can easily become the single person's weakness if they are excluded: the power of the circle is that it can include the late arrival with a single act of awareness. The new group is formed and the whole is enhanced by the additional member.

Cycles and circles

Our time frame encourages us to think in terms of time being linear, but the symbolism of the circle is quite apparent in our language. We talk of the cycles of the seasons, the life-cycle, and the cycle of day and night. The movement of the Earth and Moon creates our months, days and years. We can envisage a set of concentric circles, the inner one represents day and night; it is surrounded by the weekly cycle; then the monthly; then the seasonal; finally we see the yearly cycle.

Is that really the end? What about the cycle of life and rebirth? As with the circle there is no end; each cycle is a macrocosm of the previous one and a microcosm of the next. We are inevitably caught up in the circularity of life, yet we often do not recognise it or its importance.

The circle has been used to depict this cyclical nature in many ways: the signs of the zodiac are drawn in a circle, and the symbol for the Earth is a cross within a circle; Jung's life cycle is drawn in circular form divided into four quarters representing birth/childhood, youth/young adulthood, mature adulthood, and old age/death. The same symbol of cross within circle can be used to illustrate the cycle of the seasons.

Nature is abundant with examples of this symbolic form: our eyes are circular; we see a circular horizon; the spiral of the snail is based on arcs of circles; most flowers have a circularity and their petals are arranged in spirals (which I see as moving circles). In fact very little in Nature is in straight lines, from the trunks and branches of trees, to the dome of the sky above us. In the Spring I love to see the bracken poking through the ground: it pushes up with its 'head' in a spiral shape, presumably this makes it stronger in its journey to the surface. It then slowly unfurls when it has reached the light. On our pond, the lily pads are circular and so are the water snails' eggs laid underneath them. The leaves of alternate-leaved plants are attached to the stem in a spiral pattern. Circles and spirals are in evidence wherever I look.

So when we dance in a circle we reflect the reality of Nature around us. We dance the symbol of our life and our existence.

"Recognising the cycles of the seasons you are able to recognise the cycles in your own life. Bringing the mind and body in harmony with the cycles of Nature allows you to experience the changes in your own body, in your feelings, your emotions and your reactions. The continuous cycle of birth, growth, death and rebirth is reflected in every aspect of life. The end is also the beginning and the cycle starts again giving new opportunity for growth and development. The cycles are continuous, the circle always complete, the harmony ever present and the energy ever available. The circle represents wholeness, unity, healing and is the basic unit of the Universe. Energy concentrated at the centre of the circle by joining hands immediately creates a powerful impulse. Energy flowing round the circle and passing across it — the ancient symbol of the circle and the cross. Come together in the circle in harmony recognising the power of the circle and the eternal cycle of the seasons, the turning circle of the year."

I wrote this piece some years ago for a celebration of the Spring equinox. It epitomises for me the connection between the cycles of the seasons, the cycles in our lives, and the dancing circle, in which we hold in microcosm the cycles of Nature: there is no beginning and no end. We demonstrate the movement of the planets round the sun, the seasonal changes we witness and the unity of the whole. For that moment we are all these things: it could go on for ever, as do the seasons and the endless rotation of the Earth.

A favourite passage from one of the native American Indian cultures illustrates this:

> "Everything that the power of the world does is done in a circle. The sky is round and I have heard that the earth is round like a ball, so are all the stars. The wind in its greatest powers whirls. Birds make their nests in circles for theirs is the same religion as ours. The sun comes forth and goes down again in a circle, the moon does the same and both are round. Even the Seasons form a great circle when they are changing, they always come back to where they were. The life of a man is a circle from childhood and so it is in everything where power moves. Our tepees were round like the nests of birds and these were always set in a circle, the nation's hoop, a nest of many nests where the Great Spirit meant for us to hatch our children."

Some observations

The mirror-image effect

One aspect of Sacred Circle Dance that has always fascinated me is the mirror-image effect. The other side of the circle appears to be going in the opposite direction to me. In fact this can be very confusing for beginners especially if they stand on the other side of the circle from the teacher. They get a 'mirror image' and are fooled into moving in the wrong direction. This even extends to putting one foot behind the other instead of in front. When Richard and I run our workshops we stand on opposite sides of the circle so that everyone has somebody near them to watch.

From the other side of the circle it appears as though I am doing the exact opposite of what I am asking them to do. Is this effect symbolic I wonder? How often in life does it feel as though people are moving in exactly the opposite direction? If we look at it again we may find that they are just in a different position on the 'circle of life'; not in front or behind but different. We can become more tolerant of each other's foibles and actions if we think like this.

Out of synch

In many of the Balkan dances the phrasing of the movements is different from that of the music. It feels as though the dance is cutting across the tune. Again I think this is highly symbolic. I expect most of us have found in everyday life that it feels as though we are 'dancing to a different drummer' from the rest of humanity. Everything seems to be out of phase and we question whether we are wrong ourselves. Yet at the end of the dance the music and movement are once more in synchronicity. So too we can find that we come back into rhythm in our lives.

Maybe it is important to allow those times of being out of kilter. It can be hard to 'go against the flow' but sometimes we have to in order to preserve our integrity. We must stand up for what we believe in and continue to dance our own dance. If we are right, maybe others will join us.

Sometimes we find ourselves dancing to the rhythm of material living, the noise of the world. We cannot hear the subtler rhythms of life, yet we must learn to hear and dance to them. Yes, we may seem to travel in a different direction and to a different tune to other people, but perhaps we need to. Maybe we all have to wake up to the inner beat of the heart and travel in a new direction too.

Integrating the shadow

Over recent years we have heard a great deal about the shadow and are encouraged to investigate it, to plunge into the depths and accept those aspects of our nature that we would rather keep hidden from ourselves let alone other people. I have always been concerned about this idea: It seems easy for it to become a journey of self-inflicted pain. I believe that it is more productive to change our attitude to the present, adjust our current belief system; then the past will change too or at least our perception of it. If we look on every experience as being positive, a part of our learning here on Earth, the 'bad' memories can be seen in a different light. Now they cease to be the trauma that caused all the quirks in our character and provides us with an 'excuse' for being the way we are today. They become the building blocks on which we can create our present life, the wonderful experiences that make each of us the rich and fulfilled person we really are.

For me this is symbolised in the dancing circle. We move round a candle and, when the main lights in the hall are out, our shadows dance round behind us. The closer we move to the centre, to the light, the bigger the shadows become. So in life the more we try to seek insight and clarity, the more darkness we seem to reveal. There is hope though: if we were to enter into the light of the candle, the shadow would completely disappear. Is this what is meant by enlightenment?

Conclusion

The symbolic nature of dancing in a circle (wholeness, healing), making the same movements (unity), being equal (harmony) and getting simple enjoyment from our own efforts (freedom) seems to be the essence of Sacred Circle Dance.

Considering the symbolism in the circle has taken us beyond the simple geometrical figure and into more esoteric aspects of life. We have found in these few pages that the dances become a microcosm of other parts of life and can teach us about ourselves and our very existence in the cycles of Nature. There is so much to be learned from moving together in a circle, from our interaction with each other to the depths of our own being.

Yet it is not necessary to see the dances in this way: that is part of the joy of them. We can treat them just as an enjoyable form of exercise or as a means of discovering about ourselves. Both are equally valid and both can be accommodated in the same circle. These dances are truly international and truly inclusive. All colours of the rainbow can co-exist.

International Language of Dance

Dance has taken us to many parts of the UK and to a number of different countries. This has been a great thrill for us — we love travelling, with the difficult decisions as to what to take with us, the excitement of the airport or seaport, the actual journey and the joy of meeting other people.

Eire

In Eire, of course, we have little trouble with the language, except that some people speak very fast and I have to really concentrate to catch the words! It is a matter of tuning in. Southern Ireland is a beautiful country and we have been particularly lucky with the weather — how many people do you know who can say they spent five days on the West coast without a cloud in the sky? On our trips we run a weekend workshop and then take a short holiday to explore different parts of the country. We love it there: the people we have met are so gentle and generous, and they really enjoy the dance.

On our first visit I sat down on the opposite side of the room to Richard: we always position ourselves apart from each other in the group. This avoids the focus being directed only to one part of the circle. In discussion sessions, we become one with the group rather than being seen as 'the facilitators'. In this way, between us, we are able to observe everyone in the circle and their perceived needs. While we are dancing it avoids the mirror-image effect I mentioned previously — everyone can see one of us on their own side of the circle.

My neighbour was armed with pen and paper all ready to take notes when the 'lecture' started. She asked: "Which one is the lecturer?" I smiled and replied: "Well, it isn't actually a lecture, and I'm one of the teachers!" Very soon she found herself discarding the notepad and dancing. The format that we use is far removed from all sitting down listening to one person talking. Notes are not appropriate (unless you want to be sure of remembering the steps of a dance at a later date). How often are copious notes taken at a meeting only to be filed along with many others and never referred to again?

In our experience, the language of Sacred Circle Dance seems to transcend words: it is universal. In our workshops participants frequently have very real and personal experiences which they take home to reflect upon. We use dance instead of words and thus allow everyone to take away just what they need. Dance gives them a safe place to learn something of what makes them 'tick'.

We have explored various themes in Eire and have been struck by how Sacred Circle Dance seems to tease out the very roots of people's concerns, for instance, the situation in Northern Ireland. On our second visit to Cork, the discussion period at the end of the weekend gave an insight about the place of power and love in relation to "the troubles" in the North. In terms of the Irish question, the power demonstrated by some sections of society needs to be tempered by love: it needs to be transformed into the power of love, a love that encompasses all, not one that clings to, or favours, a particular group of people. It was this that led us to create the workshop to look specifically at these two aspects of human experience — power and love (which we discuss more fully in a later chapter). We can talk this language so easily in dance: we can act it out; we can become that love and the barriers are broken down.

Poland

Our other great love is Poland. On our second visit we travelled by coach: it was a long journey (29 hours) with only half a dozen ten-minute stops apart from the Channel crossing, so by the time we reached the East German–Polish border we were quite tired. It took about two and a half hours to get through customs and we could not see any real reason for this; there was just a huge queue waiting to get across. Finally we were in Poland and driving past numerous roadside shops selling painted garden gnomes: it was a bizarre sight, but apparently this is a Polish export to Germany!

Then an amazing thing happened: we had been in Poland for about ten minutes in a region we had not seen before, when I had an overwhelming feeling of 'coming home'. That is the only way I can describe it. I had certainly not anticipated this: I was looking forward to meeting up with friends from the previous year, but never expected to feel so emotional when we crossed the border.

I thought it was the effect of tiredness or sitting in one position for so long and I kept quiet. Soon, though, I had to express it: "I've got a really strange feeling; it's as if I have come home. I can't explain it any other way." "I'm feeling exactly the same way," said Richard. We sat looking at each other with tears in our eyes and lumps in our throats. Here we were in the far West of Poland, with unfamiliar scenes passing before our eyes and with a deep sense of returning home. What has this to do with Sacred Circle Dance? The previous year we had run workshops at a summer camp at a tiny village called Wronje (pronounced Vronyay) in the heart of Poland. We could only say 'Yes', 'No' and 'Thank you' in Polish and yet the dance had broken down the communication barriers and we had come to a deep feeling for the people and their culture.

We had a translator for the descriptive parts of the workshops, but the dance spoke for itself. I found that the best way to teach in these circumstances was to dance in the centre of the circle and for the group to copy my movements. In fact this is probably a more effective way to learn than with a lot of words, because the body, not the head, learns the dance. I often say when I am teaching that it is a good idea to tell yourself, "I have no head!". I demonstrate that I can see the whole of my body from the tips of my toes all the way up to my shoulders, and then it stops — I cannot see my head. This is how it can be in Sacred Dance: my body moves with the circle, in time with the music, but my head, my mind, is not involved. I just experience the motion, the emotion, the essence of the dance, and I am renewed.

The body is an effective tool for remembering movements. If *it* knows the dance, when the music is played it will recall the steps and how it danced them before.

When someone is having difficulty getting the steps right, they will often mentally 'give up': they resign themselves to not being able to do this dance. Then, as if by some miracle, they are doing it correctly. Yet it is no miracle: it seems that the body has heaved a sigh of relief because the head is no longer interfering, trying to get it right, and failing dismally. It is the body that moves, the body that creates the beautiful patterns, and the body that will do this again another day. The head, the brain, has little part to play, and is best taking a back seat.

Our experience in Poland of teaching by demonstration, made us realise very forcefully what an international language Sacred Circle Dance is. We tell each other a great deal about ourselves by the way we move, the ease or otherwise of dancing the steps, and the expression we bring to the movements. We move in harmony without the need for words. Dancing together, we know each other at a level deeper than any words can convey. In the circle we share a common intention, which is hard to achieve with words, as the diplomats and policy-makers of the world know only too well. I have a dream that if all the leaders of the world would only dance together there would be no wars.

We have now started learning Polish — and that is not easy. When we went there in 1996, I taught the dances in their own language. This was naturally very well received because they are aware of how difficult it is for us to even pronounce some of their words let alone remember them! It made the teaching flow much better, but I was still aware of the power of the dance to surmount these artificial barriers of language. At the end of the day we are all human beings with remarkably similar fears, pleasures and hopes whatever language we speak and whatever the differences in our culture. This is emphasised when we join hands and dance together.

Israel

We arrived in Tel Aviv the day after the assassination of Yitzhak Rabin. The night before we had already gone to bed, ready for an early start the next morning. The telephone rang and Richard's parents broke the stunning news. Would we be allowed into Israel? Would our friends be able to get to the airport to meet us? We went to sleep that night with these and many other questions going round and round in our minds. As it turned out, we were close to the last flight that was allowed to land at Tel Aviv the following day. Soon after we touched down the airport was closed to the public ready for the arrival of the dignitaries.

What an experience it was to be there that week. We are convinced that it was no coincidence that we had chosen that time to go: we had had an open invitation to visit our friends and had picked this particular week. We shared in the grief of the people, we witnessed their bewilderment and we felt a deep closeness with them in their loss and confusion. We went to the square, now called Yitzhak Rabin Square, filled with people on a vigil and lit by thousands of candles, some in long lines, some in the most exquisite patterns like a garden of light. With awe we realised the quietness, the peace, that pervaded among a crowd of thousands. There was no music, no loud voices, only a quiet, gentle hush.

A very poignant moment for us was seeing a young man in his early twenties in army uniform. He moved along the column of candlelight with his companion, another soldier. He bent down to light his own candle to add to the tribute. He only had one leg. It touched us deeply.

When we planned our trip we had hoped to visit a number of groups to learn new Israeli dances, which are great favourites of ours. The circumstances of our visit made this impossible because no groups were meeting that week: it would have been disrespectful and besides nobody had the heart to dance. In the end Dahlia, our hostess, taught us four simple dances in her tiny kitchen: she played the music on an accordion while we recorded her. It is a real joy and a wonderful memory to dance those dances now, with the 'live' music, and be transported back to their flat in the centre of Tel Aviv.

We were due to run two mini-workshops based on 'Dancing the Sevenfold Energies of Life' (described in detail later), which our friend Arnon had organised for us. He is a lecturer in humanistic psychology and we were to take his Monday afternoon and Wednesday morning groups. The former was a collection of primary school teachers and the latter a group of volunteers who were training in various aspects of emergency/crisis work. Dancing was to be a very different means of learning for them from the usual lecture format and there was a certain amount of excitement and anticipation in the air despite the circumstances.

It was made very clear at the start that the dancing we were leading was an educational exercise and that this was in no way a social occasion. We were all there to explore our own personalities. The session with the voluntary crisis workers had started late because it had rained while we were driving from Tel Aviv to Haifa. This might not sound very significant, but in Israel it is like snow in England: everything stops! There are no gullies at the side of the roads (well rain is a rarity) so the water builds up and the road floods. It rained hard too, so the mud was being washed off the fields onto the road and chaos ensued.

Eventually we arrived, a little harassed but otherwise none the worse for wear. They were a wonderful group of caring, concerned people. We had purposely not used any Israeli dances because, if by any chance they had reached me not in their original form, a discussion about the 'right' steps or emphasis might detract from the learning process. They found some of the dances difficult but were prepared to explore why that might have been. At the end we had a long discussion about the nature of the dance and what it had conveyed to them. Once again the international language of dance was apparent.

The questions raised as a result of the direct and immediate experience of the dance were searching to say the least. The most poignant, from one of the women, really seemed to sum up the feeling of the group and certainly hit home with us: "How can we get away from the fanaticism and conflict and live our lives with love and wisdom?". It came direct from her heart, brought up by the horror of the last few days and the fear of the future. At the end of the ensuing discussion someone said, "Maybe dance is the answer — to all dance together without restriction of race or creed". This would certainly be a powerful tool in the peacemakers' kit, and a universal language to speak.

Interestingly enough, many of the Israeli dances are very gentle. The music is exquisite and can move people to tears. Yet the Jewish nation has lived through one conflict after another, and survives through its strength of will. In the cafés, in their homes and in Yitzhak Rabin Square we experienced a very tender people, who were more bewildered than angry, who still long for the day when they may live in peace with themselves and their neighbours.

We were proudly taken to the Jordanian border where we would have been in fear of sniper fire only so recently. When we were there all was quiet and you would never have known the tensions that had existed.

To show the effect of dance, since we came back from Israel, our hosts have used their own Israeli dances in much the same way as we do. Our short workshops gave them an insight into how dance can be a means of getting to know more about ourselves and each other. It brings an immediate, forceful and direct experience: it transcends the artificial boundaries of language and country.

The power of dance

At the end of our fortnight of workshops in Poland in 1997, Grenardy, one of the participants, told us a story:

"A well-known Jewish Rabbi was to visit a small Russian village. The populace was excited and full of anticipation. They
had spent weeks deciding what questions they would ask the
great man. The day dawned and the nervousness and apprehen-
sion were almost tangible.

The synagogue was full: not a spare seat was to be seen.
The Rabbi arrived and the congregation waited in hushed ex-
pectancy. Their honoured guest sat quietly for some time and
then he started to hum. The people joined in and the tension
began to be broken. He sang a song and they all joined in, enjoying the involvement. Finally he got up and danced and the
congregation left their seats and followed him. When they were
all exhausted and exhilarated, the Rabbi sat down again and said
quietly to the assembled crowd: "I hope I have answered all
your questions!"

He walked out of the synagogue and everyone agreed that it
had been a most rewarding and fulfilling experience. All the
questions they would have put to him had gone out of their heads:
they no longer needed the answers."

As he told the story I felt it was describing what he had experienced in the
dancing. What was so wonderful for me is that this story is an old favourite of mine, one I have used on many occasions to illustrate the power of
dance. On the other side of Europe we hear the same tale, and the only
difference is that it happened in a Russian village, not an Israeli one!

Getting to Know Other Cultures

Before I started Sacred Circle Dancing I knew little about the other cultures around the world. Through dancing to their music and experiencing
the effect on me and other people, I feel a certain empathy with the many
countries from which the dances originate. In addition, I have picked up
snippets of information from other teachers about the cultures, the history of the people and the type of life they lead. This is all important
background to the dances themselves: it helps us to understand, and feel
closer to, the nations whose dances we use, even if we have not visited
the countries ourselves.

Romania

A radio programme soon after the downfall of Ceausescu moved me deeply. It told of the restrictions that had been placed on the people during his 'rule': they were apparently not allowed to do their own dances or sing their own songs. It described how the folk tradition was actively destroyed; many villages were razed to the ground and replaced by blocks of flats. It left me wondering whether there are enough people still alive in Romania who know the dances of their own tradition to be able to pass them on to the younger generation. Indeed do the young people want to learn them and retain their folk roots? Perhaps the dances of the Circle Dance movement hold the key to a forgotten heritage. I do know that it is important for me to continue to dance them and pass them on.

Generally the steps of these dances are intricate; the music and the movements tend to be lively and somewhat vigorous. They make me feel good, they invoke in me a sense of fun, the joy and excitement of meeting together to dance. Alunelul (meaning Little Hazelnut), for instance, is a great favourite: it is basically a simple dance but it is deceiving — it is easy to go wrong! We only have to count up to three, yet that can be extraordinarily difficult sometimes. At the end of each sequence we stamp, as a result of which it is often called the nutcracker dance. I have a lovely picture of people wearing shoes that are like clogs, breaking nuts by stamping on them.

Lamiita is an interesting dance. It is fast, so can be tiring. Yet, if we lean out as we whirl round, the circle gains its own momentum and it as if we are flying. We use the structure of the circle to give us energy. It needs everybody in the group to participate fully though, otherwise the circle is pulled in one direction and loses its form. For me this is a really important aspect of these dances: they are an expression of true community, in which all are needed and all play a part in creating the whole. At the end we feel a little breathless but very energised and at one with each other.

In contrast, there is a beautiful bride's dance, Hora de Miressi, which tells us some of the old Romanian tradition. It is slow, very pensive, and rather sad with a number of hesitations and changes of direction. I find myself thinking of arranged marriages, when the newly married girl went to her husband's home to look after him and his family, and rarely saw her own family or friends. This feels like a dance of farewell to the old life: a time of deep reflection, uncertainty and even fear. It is incredibly moving.

Most of the Romanian dances I know have a real feeling of celebration about them. I find myself reflecting on the terrible stories we have heard of the orphanages in Romania and how sharp is the contrast between the plight of those children and the exciting and carefree nature of the dances. I suppose all countries have these contrasts but it is brought into strong focus for me through the dances.

Bulgaria

We went to a wonderful evening of Bulgarian singing, dancing and music a few years ago in Winchester. The Bisserov sisters and their musicians have an incredible musical talent. Of course they were dressed in national costume which brought the dances to life. It must be so different wearing such beautiful clothes: they seem to give a poise, strength and elegance which our modern western clothes lack.

They taught us a beautiful simple dance that I could have danced all evening. It apparently fitted many of the Bulgarian tunes and we danced it whenever we could. They demonstrated their instruments and at the break we had an opportunity to 'have a go'. The drums were particularly fascinating to us; they produced a deep, powerful resonance that seemed to echo progressively across the hall. They also played wind instruments and a type of fiddle.

The singing was a joy to listen to. We have also seen a Bulgarian choir on television and it fascinates me how they create the effect. It comes from way back in the throat, yet it sounds nasal. It is a very different way of singing from what I am used to. It produces a haunting, emotional sound. I feel that, were I to try it, I would soon have a sore throat, yet for our Bulgarian friends it is the way they sing, they have been brought up that way, and it is effortless.

During the evening in Winchester we were serenaded by these wonderful singers and transported to a different land. At the end of the evening it was difficult to believe that we were still here in England. We had really experienced a few hours of another culture: we had heard how the instruments are made; we had danced traditional dances to live Bulgarian music; we had been a part of the songs; and we felt great empathy with these lovely women and their homeland.

For me there is an elegance about Bulgarian dances which reflects how I felt about the costumes the Bisserov sisters wore. Mari Mariko, danced with a certain precision, makes me feel strong and upright; I have to be wholly present and it is a good place to be. At the end it as if I have grown a couple of inches: I am proud to be me.

Some of the rhythms we dance to are very different from our own music; they can give a feeling of mystery which can be quite hypnotic.

I am thinking of Neda Voda Nalivala: the steps are apparently straightforward — or are they? There is a tantalising hesitation towards the end of the musical phrase before we do a quick forward and back into the centre of the circle. It is fractional and yet so poignant, like a tiny intake of breath in the dance. It is all in the rhythm of the tune which is 11/8 time. We even pause before we start to move, as if contemplating the next step. For me it shows a control, a deliberation which feels quite different from the rush and bustle, the acting without thinking which I associate with western culture.

Armenia

Very few of the Armenian dances we do will have come directly from the country itself. Armenia was, until very recently, extremely closed off from the rest of the world. We are lucky that there are large Armenian communities in other countries, such as America, Greece and the UK, and they retain their own folk traditions from the 'old country'. From them we have learned some beautiful dances and a little of their culture.

The rhythms and instruments sound different from our western music. Is this what makes the dances so fascinating to me? At the beginning of Harsaneek there is a wailing instrument that creates a wonderful atmosphere: it is haunting, almost eerie in its sound, yet it has a beauty and depth. With rhythms like long, short, medium we again come across the feeling of flow and hesitation intermingling. It seems to me to reflect life: at times we move forward, at others we have to stop and reassess. It is so clear in the rhythm of their music, while, in contrast, our 4/4, 3/4 rhythms do not allow us those moments of recollection and regeneration.

I have recently come across a couple of candle dances from Armenia. They introduce a new facet for me with the patterns of the lights as we progress round the circle, in and out, with the hands moving in relation to the feet as well. There is an intricacy within the simplicity: a contradiction maybe, but nevertheless a truth for me. Candlelight is so gentle, it is breathtaking to look round the group and see the beauty of each individual face. For me these dances express bringing light into darkness, our own light. We no longer rely on the external light at the centre of the circle; we have our own light to take forth into the world. This seems to be very significant in a land which has been a mystery to me for so long and which only recently has suffered earthquake and consequent disaster. Amidst all this I feel a beauty and a dignity from the dances of these people.

Russia

The Russian dances have a notable characteristic. There is a step called the Russian glide; well, it is not so much a step as a way of moving. The head stays still in relation to the floor and all the movement comes from the hips, knees and ankles. We each have to imagine we are carrying a plate on our head and not going to drop it! This is often accompanied by quite lively music. It seems to me to indicate a nation that is determined to hold its head up, to remain dignified whatever may befall. Perhaps a nation that wants to have fun but can never quite let go enough.

An example of this is Tropotianska. The tune is bright and cheerful, yet we move round the circle doing slip steps trying to keep our heads still. All our instincts make us want to free ourselves of this restriction and allow our bodies to reflect the nature of the music. There is another lesson for me in this. I could become very frustrated and rail against the lack of freedom. However, if I flow with it there is a dignity about the movement and I retain my own integrity. It fascinates me how the dances can teach us so much about life, and so graphically.

It is a very interesting experience to dance in this way: most of us in the West find it quite difficult to maintain that poise. We want to bob up and down and really express ourselves as the music seems to require. Yet we try to keep our head steady and end up feeling restricted. Thus we learn about the people whose dances we use, and about ourselves.

In the Russian weaving dances we seem to tie ourselves in knots only to unwind again and return to the normal circle. All this is done holding hands and moving under each other's arms. It is a fascinating process. While in the knot we may feel restricted and yet there is a close companionship, a feeling of "we're all in this together!". Is this reflecting the life in Russia? Does it teach us, if only a little, how it has felt to live first under the Tsars and then under another form of totalitarian rule? I certainly feel I know more about the Russian people through their dances.

Former Yugoslavia

When I ran a day of dances from former Yugoslavia to raise money for aid in Bosnia, I tried to find out which of the new states they came from. In many cases this proved difficult: we have been so used to saying that a dance is from Yugoslavia that its exact place of origin seems to have been lost. However, one thing struck me quite forcibly: I know a lot of Serbian and Macedonian dances, a few Croatian but I think only one Bosnian one. Does this tell us something of these different peoples, or is it just coincidence?

To prepare for this particular day I had visited a friend who is from former Yugoslavia: through her I had found out a great deal of information about the meanings of the titles of the dances. I drew a map indicating the new states, the major towns and the places of origin of some of the dances. This was greatly appreciated because we rarely stop to think how surrounded former Yugoslavia is by other nations: how must it feel to have seven countries bordering your own? Are border disputes inevitable? The feeling around the circle on that day was one of constriction, as if, in that situation, we would feel a need to protect ourselves continually, just in case… Seeing the geography of the region seemed to enhance the experience of the day and invoked a very personal reaction to the Yugoslavian situation.

The dances and the small amount of material I had put together about them had brought us closer to the people of former Yugoslavia in their terrible plight. There was a tremendous atmosphere of empathy. Somehow we had transcended the artificial political boundaries and were united in the dance.

Greece

In the dances from Greece we again face the challenge of unusual rhythms: some people struggle to get their mind or feet round a tune with seven, nine, eleven and even thirteen beats to the bar. Seven beats to the bar we can think of as long, short, short (or dactylic); nine beats to the bar can be thought of as long, short, shorter! But it gets somewhat complex if we try to extend this any further. In fact it is much more complicated to consider it at a theoretical level than it is to just do the dances. Again we come back to letting our head take a back seat and allowing the body to move in time with the music.

These rhythms have a beauty all of their own and remind me of sun-drenched beaches, sitting in the taverna drinking coffee, eating yogurt and honey, and just lazing around. In the rhythm and the style of the music I am transported into a holiday atmosphere.

When celebrating a season of the year, a number of the dances I choose are from Greece, perhaps because they are used for this same purpose in their country of origin. Many of them are closely related to celebration of the agricultural cycle or mark significant times in individual or community life.

The dances themselves tend to be danced facing the centre; they are fairly precise even when they are fast. In Greece the way the feet are lifted in a simple dance like Servico, which consists of side, behind, side, lift, side, lift, is quite exact. When I was on Skopelos some years ago I was particularly struck with the way these lifts were executed. In the first one the left leg came across the right with the heel leading; in the second the right foot was just brought to the side of the left. In this country I think we tend to dance in a much less accurate style.

I experience a certain formality in the dances, and yet they generate a tremendous sense of connectedness. Originally most of them would have been done in a shoulder hold: this has become rather corrupted here because, not being used to holding our arms in this position for a long time, we find it very tiring. We often adjust it to holding the hands at shoulder height but not actually on the shoulders of our neighbours. Nevertheless, we retain some of the closeness and this can give a powerful feeling of unity of purpose and a strong sense of comradeship.

The Greek dances speak of a great community atmosphere: it may be enhanced by ouzo and retsina but it is the whole village celebrating. Well, that is not strictly true, because, although I have seen younger women joining in, it seems that it is usually only the men that dance, in public at least. What a difference from our western culture where the men often have to be dragged kicking and screaming onto the dance floor!

Macedonia

For many years I had a real problem with Macedonian dances. I had a vision of them being aggressive, warlike and very masculine. I did not teach them and rarely danced them in other circles. Finally I decided I had to get over this feeling of antagonism and I started introducing a few into my repertoire. Now I find it difficult to believe that I ever felt like I did, because, as soon as I let go of my resistance, exquisite, gentle dances came my way. Legnala Dana, for instance, became my favourite dance for a long time (actually that is difficult to define because they are all my favourite dance!). In this we come back to the long, short, short rhythm and we seem to move effortlessly round: the atmosphere of the music is peaceful, positive and in sharp contrast to my previous vision of Macedonian dances.

Then there are fast and invigorating dances such as Ekislisko Horo. We 'fly' into the centre and out again making a 'slice of cake' pattern on the floor, and we retrace our steps. As the music speeds up it feels as though a wind is blowing through my hair. The dance ends with a determined three stamps, which when done in unison is very satisfying. I find this quite hypnotic; I want it to go on for ever, yet at the end, whilst being energised, I am also exhausted. Time for a slow dance to bring the group down and back to 'normality'. There is a certain sense of chaos in this dance and at the same time a determination. It is not aggressive like the dances I struggled with earlier, yet it reaches its goal in a very focused manner.

Macedonia has a history of being part of many other countries and the variety I have now found in the dances seems to bring this out. Yes, there is the warlike aspect brought about by the situation the people have found themselves in. Yet there is also the gentle, nurturing face, the energetic side and the dogged persistence to their nature.

Costume

When teaching women's dances from the Balkan region I emphasise the style of the steps, which is small with tiny lifts, unlike our western movements. This is because of the weight of the costumes that the women wear: it would be difficult to take a large step to either side or lift the leg very high. This was really brought home to me when we went to an exhibition of Balkan costume at the Museum of Mankind in London. There we saw a Macedonian girl's wedding dress festooned with metal discs of decoration. The text beside it said that it weighed a hundredweight (nearly 51 kgs)! Imagine carrying that around all day, even if it was only for one occasion. The truth of the woman's situation was suddenly real and I knew, as I had not done before, how difficult it would be to move.

There is a grace about taking these small steps and only lifting the foot an inch off the ground. It is much more elegant than the large steps that are our normal way of travelling. Somehow our movements become gross in comparison. Yet think of the restriction that the women must feel in these countries when wearing their national costume. I am fascinated how difficult people find it in the West to make these tiny movements: I suppose we have been 'free' of long, heavy dresses for so long that we have lost that precision and elegance. Doing dances of which this is a feature brings back a lost part of myself: I can feel myself change as mentally I attempt to put myself into someone else's shoes (and clothes). My poise and balance increase and I begin to feel graceful.

Israel

Israeli dances are mostly recent choreographies since the creation of the state of Israel in 1949, yet they have their roots in the Jewish communities all round the world. Many Israelis have 'returned' to Israel from the

East European countries where they considered themselves in exile. They have taken with them the culture they were surrounded by and thus influenced the dances. When asked if English is still the second language in Israel, our Jewish friend replied with a smile, "No, Hebrew is the second language; Russian is the first!".

There are many Israeli dances which tell the story of finding a homeland. This is a recurring theme and the steps create something of a wistful atmosphere, a yearning for a stable place to live. They speak of a hunger for peace, for a home and for an 'ordinary' life of tilling the fields and tending the grapevines.

Songs like Rakud ha Shalom speak of the bravery of those who fought in the Six Day's War and of the horrors of war. The first verse ends with the words:

> I give you my promise, my dear little girl,
> That this will be the very last war.

One of my favourite Israeli dances is Omrim Yeshna Eretz. The song is about a beautiful place:

> They say there is a land
> A land of bountiful sun
> Where is such a land and such a sun?
> They say there is a land,
> Her pillars are seven,
> And seven her guiding stars...
> This land for which all hope
> Does indeed exist...

In Hora Galile (or "Let's build the Galilee"), we are in shoulder hold, representing the concept of true community. In this position we have to move together, work together to a common purpose. Initially we just sway to the music, gathering our energy, then as the music speeds up we move in unison to a simple sequence of steps. Finally we come back to the swaying. The whole dance leaves me with a wonderful feeling of having created something beautiful — in the song it is the Galilee, and if you have been there you will understand the passion behind the dance to build a future there.

There is a wonderful range of Israeli dances; the music is often very emotive; the rhythms are familiar, often four beats to the bar, and easy for us to assimilate and understand. The dances flow effortlessly once the sequence of steps is mastered. They are often complicated but rarely difficult — the actual steps are simple while the way they are combined or the length of the phrases may be more complex.

So I have a vision of a race of people anxious to obtain stability, to find a place they can call their own, both at the level of a house and land, and of a country. This seeking has been a part of their life for many centuries and I feel privileged to share in it in dance. It serves to remind me of the pleasure I have in my home, my garden and my space around me: I try not to take it all for granted.

Iran

I only know one Iranian Circle Dance yet that one dance has allowed me a touching insight into this country. We were at the Ockenden Venture, an organisation which assists refugees from all over the world. I had been asked to lead an afternoon of dancing outside in the grounds of their lovely house in Haslemere. I knew that they had a family of Kurds from Iran so I took the tape of Khan Amiry with me. This is a dance which most people here find very difficult. The main movement is to hop on the right leg while moving the left leg out and in from the hip with the knee held high. It is tiring to say the least.

However, we never did that dance on this occasion because as soon as I played the music the father of the Kurdish family started dancing: he grabbed hold of my hand and led me round the lawn in a set of simple steps but with such elegance. There were bounces and shimmies and an atmosphere of great excitement. The line lengthened as more people joined in. No words were used — he had little English — we learned by doing, which is the natural way. Through his eldest son he told us later that there are five variations including the basic dance: he taught us the first two.

Previously this father of five had been quiet and withdrawn: the dance brought him to life. It was a moving and memorable experience. In Iran the father is very much the head of the family: in his circumstances over here, he had to bow to his sons, and even daughters, because they were picking up the language and he was struggling with it. In the dance he was again the leader, the one who showed others what to do. He was again proud, dignified and his family honoured him. By popular request he led the dance again later on in the afternoon and demonstrated his prowess.

This story becomes all the more moving when I tell you that he had left Iran, fortunately with his family, but after having been tortured — on his feet. He had difficulty walking yet the music had inspired him, his physical and emotional pain forgotten for a moment, the moment of the dance. This occasion will live on in my memory. He was an inspiration to us all with his agility, joy and strength.

Conclusion

I believe it is very important in this strife-torn world to get to know other people and other cultures. It is probably impossible to know someone from every country of the world, but through these dances we can learn something of the nature of many of the communities. I feel closer to them as I dance; I can enter a little into their world and maybe understand them a little better. I allow some of their world to enter into me, thereby making a common connection and transcending outer differences. In the end I feel that we are not so different from each other, and we can unite in the common language of dance. As I typed that sentence the word 'unite' came out as 'untie'! Maybe that is the solution — we have to 'untie the knots' we have created that prevent us from getting to know each other, from realising that we are all at heart much the same, and we are all citizens of the same planet.

Part 3

The Seven Rays

by Richard

*Acquiring my first Alice Bailey book was a turning point:
through her philosophy I was introduced to the Seven Rays,
that magnificent concept of creation having a sevenfold nature*

A Sevenfold View of Life

We are all unique and individual, but why are we comfortable with some people and not with others? Often we meet those with whom we find it difficult to conjure up any kind of rapport. Then there are some with whom we have a good relationship without any effort whatsoever. It is as though there is something that either instantly clashes or harmonises, a factor that operates distinct from our conscious awareness.

I have found Alice Bailey's concept of the Seven Rays, with its emphasis on a basic sevenfoldness in nature, helps me make sense of relationships. This is not something new to human experience. We are constantly conditioned by sevenfoldness in many common areas of life, though we rarely stop to think about them as having some deeper significance:

time — the seven days of the week;
light — the seven colours of the rainbow;
sound — the seven notes of the (western) musical scale.

Others might wish to add the following to this list:

space — the seven planes of being;
energy — the seven chakras.

Seven great streams of energy are said to pervade the whole of creation. Each stream, or Ray, carries certain essential qualities which find expression through form. Together they interweave to create the richness and diversity that we experience in our world.

What do we mean by a Ray? Essentially we are talking about a stream of energy, a vibration. Our model recognises seven such Rays, seven qualities of energy, seven differentiations of living substance which find expression through the many aspects of creation — human beings, other realms of nature, the planets and constellations. So the whole of creation is the product of these interweaving Ray energies.

'Energy' is a term that has a particular scientific application and meaning and is seen as something measurable. I use the word energy in relation to the Rays to indicate subtle influences that impinge on our natures, that provide the basis of human experience and expression. We all exist within an ocean of energy. We are ourselves systems of energy. Perhaps one day we will have instrumentation that in some way will measure Ray energy reliably. For the present, though, we measure it through human experience. By developing greater self-awareness and sensitivity to our own processes, we can differentiate between the subtle influences that shape us and induce certain characteristics in our individual and collective ways of being. We can learn how to modify and adapt these energies to enrich our creativity and effectiveness in our daily lives.

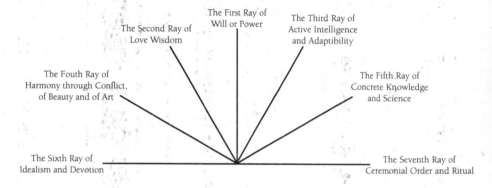

Figure 2. The Seven Rays

The names given to the Rays provide us with clues as to their nature as shown in Figure 2. They break down into seven essential types of person:[10]

- The first Ray type is likely to be a leader by inclination, often with clarity of vision and purpose. There may be a tendency to enjoy power and to exert a dominant will.
- The second Ray predisposes us towards a gentle and loving nature, to a willingness to serve, heal and placate, rather than assert the self. It can cause extreme sensitivity to the point of fearfulness.
- The third Ray type is an active person who is likely to be always busy, who is practical and efficient on material levels, intelligent and capable. This type can find it difficult to remain still.
- The fourth Ray with its dualistic process of seeking harmony through conflict, tends to produce sensitive and imaginative people with much creative potential, alongside the awareness and problems of the artistic temperament. Artistic expression, however, can be found linked to all the Rays.
- The fifth Ray stimulates the world of science and knowledge, and those who are influenced strongly by it are intellectually focused, inquiring,

---

10.   Much of this list has been taken from *The Seven Rays* (Sundial House, Tunbridge Wells).

analytical and critical, happiest when they are living entirely in their minds. It may also generate a narrowness of thought.

- The sixth Ray generates devotion and tends to produce the dedicated believer and mystic, the devotee, the idealist and, *in extremis*, the one-pointed fanatic. This energy can be applied to any ideal, not necessarily religious.
- The seventh Ray brings a great love of order and an ability to organise and relate to others. Those governed by this energy have an appreciation of law and are much concerned with form and formulation, group methods and processes. Too much order can strangle spontaneity and creativity.

The Rays and the individual

We are all affected by the energies of the Rays. Our physical/etheric bodies, emotions and minds are conditioned by Ray quality. I believe that we are more than a chemical soup contained and constrained within a physical body. Increasingly, people are investigating and accepting the existence of more subtle fields of energy. Scientifically we know we have an electromagnetic field surrounding and penetrating us. This we can measure. Why not further fields that stretch beyond the sensitivity of our physical means of measurement?

Alice Bailey's model suggests that for the most part we can expect our physical natures to be governed by either third or seventh Ray influence; our emotions by second or sixth Ray influence and our minds by first, fourth or fifth Ray influence. This is at least a starting point when we are seeking to gain insight into which energies govern our nature.

However, at certain stages on the spiritual path of development we may find ourselves with other Ray combinations. This is generally to enable an individual to work through a particular stage of growth. Bear in mind that evolutionary development as far as we are concerned is about demonstrating within ourselves an ability to master our use of force and energy, and to direct it in a wise and intelligent manner. Human beings are surely a life form that brings self-consciousness into contact with energy, leaving us with a certain freedom to choose how we will direct that energy into expression. Most of the time we do not think of this. We live habitual lives, often conditioned by what we have learned from others. And yet, even in this we will each have our own individual style. The more we reflect on ourselves, on how and who we are, the more we gain insight into the qualities that are present, or lacking, in our make-up.

There comes a point in our development when the physical/etheric, emotional and mental fields or bodies integrate into a unit that we might call the 'personality'. The individual moves beyond being subject to the different bodies pulling in different directions and, in this state, can be extremely powerful (Figure 3). The personality Ray begins to exert a strong influence and the individual develops an identity with this new, potent stream of energy. It can lead the person to change their style of living, their focus of interest or their way of functioning.

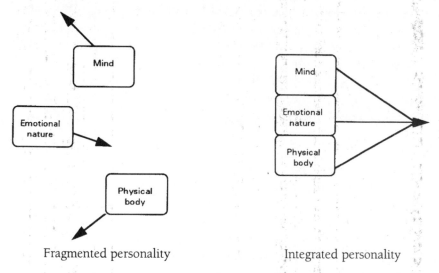

Fragmented personality   Integrated personality

Figure 3. Integration of the personality

Beyond this, and at a much deeper and subtler level, lies the Soul, which is also distinctively qualified by Ray energy. Whilst the personality can be extremely separative, the Soul is inclusive. For many people on the spiritual path their major struggle lies in reconciling the Soul and personality Rays.

The focus of our consciousness is an important factor in determining how we express Ray energy. For instance, when there is little sensitivity to the Soul we would not expect to find the Soul Ray to be a dominant feature in that person's life. Then there are individuals who are so focused in one aspect of their personality nature — the emotions, for instance — that the Rays of the mind or body may find little opportunity for expression. Those for whom the world of thought is the major focus, may well find their mental Ray dominating. Someone else may have a consciousness strongly fused with the Soul, enabling their Soul Ray to find expression through a life of service.

How do we get a sense of our Ray energies?

The simplest way to look at the Rays is in the context of your own life experience. For instance, ask yourself a few questions: Are you drawn to distinctive ways of working with people? Do you have a dominant quality or aptitude? Are there specific qualities which you feel you lack, perhaps present in fantasy but not in daily life? It can be just as important to know which energies you are not working with as it is to know those with which you are.

Take a moment to look back over your life. Has it seemed a constant struggle through conflict? Are you more comfortable when there is order? Has it got to be your order, or are you easily adaptable to other people's dictates? Is this adaptability comfortable, or are you more subservient to others, unable to voice your needs? Do you have a real issue over attention to detail? Have you devoted a lot of energy in the pursuit of some ideal? These are the sort of questions that can start us on a path towards seeing our lives in the light of the Rays.

The issue of order may be linked to the seventh Ray, but if that order involves harmony in colour and tone then fourth Ray energy may be indicated. A life-trend of struggle might also suggest the working into expression of this latter energy. Concern over detail and accuracy, particularly when thought is involved, would suggest fifth Ray influence. The ability to be adaptable could indicate the presence of the third Ray, whilst if you feel unable to stand up for yourself, fearful of being rejected if you do, then second Ray over-sensitivity could be an influence. The presence of a strong note of idealism can be linked to the sixth Ray.

I believe that taking the Rays as a psychological model and testing it against our experience is the best way to gain knowledge. There are those who claim to be able to tell you what your Rays are through various means. They may be right, they may not be. I cannot make judgements. It is their way; it is not mine. I do believe, however, that we do not need to dress the Rays up in a cloak of mystery as if knowledge of our Rays is an indication of spiritual growth or standing on the Path. It is useful knowledge and the proof of this usefulness lies in how we use it. It can be taken as an excuse for not exhibiting certain socially acceptable behaviour. It can be seen as a way of unlocking previously hidden potential. The choice is ours. If we were talking in the language of psychology there would be no mystery or bated breath around what type we conform to. Let us keep the Rays within this type of approach to self-knowledge.

Many people find the power of dance helps them to gain insight into the Ray qualities that are present or absent within themselves. We will explore this more closely in Part 4.

Strengths and weaknesses

All the Rays have virtues and vices, strengths and weaknesses. Most of the weaknesses reflect an over-emphasis on a given Ray. We have to bear in mind that these energies interweave and 'colour' each other. It is rare to find a pure Ray type. This is something of a safeguard, because otherwise the virtues or vices of the Rays could be over-emphasised and produce what might be a dangerously unbalanced expression. This can be particularly difficult when the imbalance is expressed through a consciousness that identifies strongly with the separated self — the personality or lower nature.

It seems likely that evolution is about two things: the expansion of human consciousness and the mastery of force and energy. The effect of both is to bring us to the point at which we can become co-creators in the divine process and align ourselves with divine Will. We therefore require some balance between Ray energies and need to learn how to apply them appropriately. To achieve this we have to cultivate some degree of discriminating sensitivity in order to know ourselves and the energies with which we naturally work.

The weaknesses of the first Ray include being over-dominant, arrogant and having a lack of sensitivity towards others. They tend to be vices of excess positivity, power and assertiveness. The second Ray is opposite, its weaknesses tend to be negative: over-sensitivity, indecision, non-assertiveness, finding it all too easy to fall in love with anyone and everyone.

The first Ray is also described as the Ray of the Destroyer, the second as the Ray of the Builder. The natural, human response is to feel OK about the Builder, but the Destroyer is seen as not so good. Yet we need both. The creative cycle necessarily has both destroying and building phases. The first Ray is very much a driving force or power, the second Ray has a more inclusive and nurturing quality. When these two energies are brought into co-operative relationship, there is generated a powerful combination: the driving will of the first Ray qualified by the inclusive note of the Second Ray — a true force for good in the world.

The third Ray energy of Active Intelligence and Adaptability is often regarded as fostering cunning, scheming and manipulation, especially in the individual who is very much centred in the separated self. It can also be seen stimulating great activity in some people — the type that always has to be *doing*, with no time for *being*. For anyone, however, who wishes to work in a practical manner with matter this Ray energy is vital. But it needs grounding, otherwise all the activity may bear little fruit!

I am sure we all know someone who has fourth Ray energy influencing their life: everything seems to be a battle, a constant struggle to find harmony which, when found, all too easily melts away in the heat of another battle. Theirs can be the gifts of sensitivity and spontaneity, of inspiration and appreciation of colour and beauty. When balance cannot be maintained, difficulties such as moodiness, depression and a general ambivalence towards life can ensue.

The fifth Ray type can be extremely insular, locked into a world of intellectual thought. Yet it is a valuable and necessary quality. Could our knowledge of ourselves and of the world have developed without this important energy? Fifth Ray energy can be very structured and methodical, the energy of the person who likes to analyse and for whom thought is more important than feeling.

The person who is susceptible to sixth Ray influence may experience a wide range of qualities: a fanatical missionary zeal which at its extreme can find violent and bloody expression; a tendency towards mystical experience; or a selfless devotion to caring for others. Perhaps you have a life-experience that is full of periods of strong devotion to a cause or a philosophy, or it may find expression within the family dynamic.

Seventh Ray types like to organise and to create order. Patience and discipline are two strengths associated with this energy. It can also bring a tendency towards perfectionism on the physical level. Weaknesses tend to stem from an over-emphasis of form and order. The stickler for regulations may be expressing this energy. This Ray type can also be susceptible to superstition and to excessive fascination towards anything secret and psychic.

The Rays can help us cast a light of understanding on relationship. Imagine strongly-focused fifth and sixth Ray types meeting for the first time — the former rooted in the world of analysis and intellectual thought, the latter centred in feeling and emotion. Here we see an example of people who might be unable to relate, and through no fault of their own. Yet, given the presence of another Ray energy that may be common to both, and/or a sensitivity to the Soul that may encourage a more inclusive awareness, there may be a possibility of two very different types co-operating and bringing their diverse qualities together to serve a common purpose. Thinking of the Rays in terms of colour might be helpful here. Some will clash, others will naturally harmonise. The challenge is to be not so rooted in one Ray energy that we end up only able to relate to those with similar qualities and similar energies. In the final analysis we are all multicoloured or 'multi-rayed', with each aspect of our multi-rayed natures providing a vehicle through which the Ray of the Soul can find expression.

Applying Ray energy

My experience has been that in certain situations we can invoke the type of energy we need, even when it may not naturally form part of our nature. A good way to do this is to visualise how a particular energy might find positive expression in the situation before you. You might also spend a short time holding an intense focus on the qualities associated with a Ray energy, absorbing its note as you think and feel your way into its essence.

Some people, for example, may not feel they have much first Ray in them but when the chips are down and they need to get something done, or sound a note of leadership, they can pull this energy into expression — they get 'fired up' and blaze a way forward for others to follow.

Others might need to learn to attract second Ray energy to establish empathic rapport with another, or fourth Ray energy to strengthen themselves in the role of peacemaker when some form of conflict has broken out. A person who is naturally shy and diffident may need to draw in the energy of the sixth Ray to inspire others and to encourage them to devote themselves more fully to a given ideal or goal. In another case it may be the seventh Ray that is needed to encourage greater order or rhythm in a particular line of activity.

We can see from this why, in a group or team, it may be necessary to have people with a whole variety of different Ray qualities. It may be hard for the group to hold itself together, there could be a lot of clashes, but if members can blend together with a strong group-will towards achieving a common goal, it will have much to offer. Thinking in terms of Ray energy may be of value to those who co-ordinate groups or manage teams. It may reveal areas of over-emphasis or gaps that need filling.

In terms of group work, it is interesting to note how different Ray impulses condition the way that people form groups. For instance, the first Ray type may literally grasp whoever is available, driving them to carry out their will. The person with a strong second Ray sends out an attractive note to draw co-workers to them. The third Ray is more consciously selective, choosing those who have the necessary qualities that are felt to be needed in the group. It is a great model for making sense of how your manager or team-leader functions!

Much that has been written about the Rays tends to be difficult to relate to everyday life. This is unfortunate, because it seems to me that this is where we have to start. Look at your work situation. Look at how people behave and interact. What energies are they expressing? Is your boss dominating and insensitive? Or is s/he so caring and sensitive to what others think of him or her that nothing gets done? Are you surrounded by people forever busy, maybe in an extremely ordered and efficient way, or perhaps amidst chaos with little achievement for the effort made? Do your sales people have a missionary zeal to almost force a sale, or do they work by creating a good relationship with their client and using this as the basis for their selling technique?

You can look at your home life too. Who is dominant? Who relates well with whom? Are the tensions the result of clashing energies? Can an understanding of what may be going on in terms of Ray energy help to improve things?

Readers who are involved in counselling may wish to study the topic of the Rays further. This is a particular interest of mine and it seems to me that there is enormous scope for the Seven Ray model to be absorbed into the art and science of the counselling relationship or any other form of healing. In any situation where we are trying to make sense of our experience, or of our way of being, it is a useful model to bear in mind.

Over the years, I have found Alice Bailey's writings have helped me to shed light on my experience, offering perspectives on evolution in terms of consciousness that have enabled me to make sense of much that I see and hear about in the world. Of course, it remains an hypothesis, to be tried and tested against what I experience. We do not tend to build into our philosophy of life ideas that actually serve to confuse us. We want to make sense of our experiences; we want to gain a greater depth of understanding and, increasingly, people seem to want to become more fully conscious in their participation in the human story. An appreciation of the Seven Rays, how they affect us, how they are expressed through us and others, can serve to deepen the quality of our lives and our relationships, enabling us to move forward with greater tolerance and understanding. The Seven Ray model reinforces the idea that we are all unique, that we each have within us intriguing mixtures of energy and potential. As we move inexorably towards greater human-to-human contact on a global scale, we are challenged to embrace and celebrate difference, and to cease to feel threatened by it.

Reflections on the Life-cycle

In terms of cosmic evolution, the One Light is said to have differentiated first into three, then into seven streams of energy. All matter, energy, spirit is composed of these seven living energies which pervade the cosmos. Each has its own quality, note or nature which conditions or qualifies our individual and group ways of being.

The Seven Ray model suggests we are all, in our own way, working to express energies and to bring them under the directing influence of the Soul. Each Ray energy uniquely expresses an aspect of Life. They interact and interweave to generate the rich tapestry of expression through form and consciousness that we see in the world. All that has been created expresses Ray quality, whether we speak of the individual human being, a kingdom of nature or a nation of the world.

The first, second and third Rays, called the 'Rays of Aspect', correspond to the basic triplicity found in many spiritual traditions representing the triple nature of Deity: for instance, Father–Son–Holy Ghost; Shiva–Vishnu–Brahma. In both a symbolic and a very real sense, the first three Ray energies are the blueprint from which the created universe takes its form. The other four Rays, called the 'Rays of Attribute', provide further texture, colour and pattern within creation.

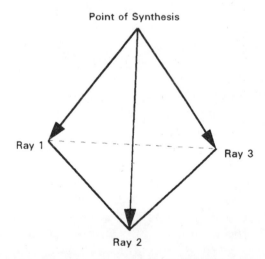

Figure 4.
The Rays of Aspect
forming a tetrahedron

We use a tetrahedron to represent the interaction of Ray energy. The apex is the point of synthesis from which the first three Rays emerge in three lines to form the points at the base of the tetrahedron (Figure 4). The four faces can then be taken to represent the other four Rays. The resulting tetrahedron (Figure 5), has the face of the fifth Ray opposite the point of the third Ray, the face of the sixth Ray opposite the point of the second Ray, the face of the seventh Ray opposite the point of the first Ray. And the base? The fourth Ray, the linking, midway energy complementing the point of synthesis.

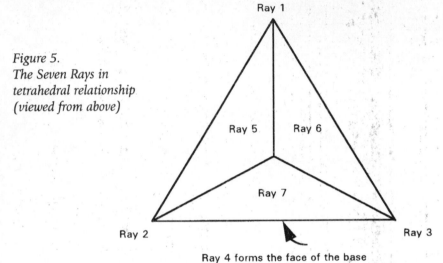

Figure 5.
The Seven Rays in
tetrahedral relationship
(viewed from above)

Ray 4 forms the face of the base

Each life is part of a greater process of spiritual development in which our individual consciousness opens up to, and becomes absorbed into, a higher state of consciousness — the Soul. The whole process of evolution from this perspective places consciousness as the primary factor. The physical, emotional and mental realms are simply the fields within and through which individual self-consciousness develops.

At a point approaching mid-life, if the necessary development has taken place, the Soul nature will begin to exert a growing influence over the developing individual consciousness leading to fusion and a staged entrance into realms of consciousness more inclusive and universal in nature.

There are exceptions, individuals for whom the Soul takes control at a much earlier age, stimulating profound thought and creativity in many forms. A number of truly visionary thinkers gained their greatest insights at an early age, a first touch of Soul upon a mechanism that is already sensitive and receptive, Einstein for instance. Child genius may also, in some cases, result from an early connection with the Soul nature, or a connection that was not broken in the process of coming into incarnation, for example, Mozart.

However, this does not mean that the connection can be maintained throughout life. Some of the great tragic figures of history are those who once knew what it was to have a mind open and alive to universal experience yet who, in later life, lost it as earthly existence and separative conditioning began to take hold.

It is also worth mentioning that many children report a sensitivity to subtle energy, to seeing colours and energy flow which most adults do not see. This is well documented and I have certainly heard children describe in an extremely matter-of-fact manner, for instance, the light they have seen passing through a room during a meditation. I sometimes wonder if part of the struggle of young people lies in their sensitivity to subtle energy and the psychological pain that is created by being forced to deny its existence. Could one result be an unconscious urge to use hallucinogenic substances to try to regain what has been lost?

Stages of the life-cycle

Each stage in the individual life-cycle involves both development and crisis. We can consider the following critical periods:

4–7 years	appropriation of the physical body
7–14 years	appropriation of the emotional body
21–25 years	appropriation of the mental body
35 years	personality prepared for the Soul
35–42 years	Soul appropriation of personality
49 years	pathway of life service should have been defined
56–63 years	decision by the Soul as to whether life will continue.

We are considering an individual spark of consciousness coming into incarnation and gradually, through the first half of life, taking a hold over the physical, emotional and mental natures. We co-ordinate and learn to direct their activity through our experiences in life. It is later, if the personality is sufficiently integrated and oriented towards the higher values, that the Soul may itself take control and 'appropriate' it as a vehicle for higher expression.

If these stages are worked through and development takes place by the age of 35, a personality mechanism will have been developed that is suitable for the Soul to work out its own purpose. It may not be rounded out, for the Soul may require some imbalance in order to fulfil certain demands that will be made upon it. It is important to differentiate here between the personality mechanism and personality consciousness. The mechanism is the integrated physical, emotional and mental natures which provides the vehicle through which the personality consciousness can gain experience and work. The goal is for the personality consciousness to become fused with that of the Soul, the mechanism then being the vehicle for *Soul-infused* expression.

These ideas are rooted in a world-view that stretches beyond the concept of there being just one life. Life is seen as a progression of lives within a continuum of rebirth which results in the development, expansion and refinement of consciousness. Each life offers the possibility of building on the achievements of previous incarnations.

The life-cycle contains a series of stages, during which the vehicles of expression are developed and brought into activity and individual consciousness is developed. So, for instance, in the early years of life the Ray of the physical vehicle will be a major factor in shaping the child's psyche. Much of the learning that will stimulate conscious growth flows from the physical environment.

Later, as the emotional vehicle develops, its Ray quality will become the primary impulse shaping the child's world of experience. If we remain with an emotional focus throughout our lives we will continue to express this energy and dwell largely in our feelings.

If our mind nature is stimulated and awakened, the Ray of the mind will come into expression. At first, our thinking will be largely shaped by emotional reactions, but in time thought itself will dominate. Our consciousness becomes more firmly established within our mental nature.

A further stage sees the integration of our personality (see Figure 3, previous chapter) with its distinctive Ray energy coming to the fore. We direct this Ray energy towards either selfish or altruistic ends, depending on where our consciousness is focused. As our consciousness continues to expand to touch the realm of the Soul, even in some small measure, we move from separateness towards universality. As the Soul's nature unfolds and our response to its influence increases, its Ray energy works through into expression in our daily life, into our sphere of service.

We might reflect on the possibility that the Soul is seeking to take a firm hold of its mechanism. There occurs "a crisis between the thirty-fifth and forty-second years, wherein conscious contact with the soul is established; the threefold personality then begins to respond, as a unit, to soul impulse".[11] This has the effect of pushing elements of the unconscious into our awareness and expanding our sense of self. We become more acutely aware of contrasts within our natures. It can be uncomfortable. Could it be the light of the Soul that breathes new life into the individual, inspiring him or her into a new direction? We may respond, we may not. We can choose — it will not be easy.

---

11.   Alice A Bailey, *Esoteric Psychology*, vol II (vol II of the five-volume *A Treatise on the Seven Rays*) (Lucis Press Ltd, London) p. 53.

Esoteric psychology suggests that these first 35 years of life are essentially a microcosm of the stages of consciousness that humanity collectively has passed through. Humanity today is faced with the struggle of being less emotionally driven and more focused in a state of mind that can reflect Soul impulse. At 35, individuals may be ready to begin to shoulder the burden of intelligent discipleship, to respond to the directing light of the Soul.

This can lead to a 'crisis of opportunity'. We have many choices to make between the ages of 25 and 40 relating to our life's work, place of living and relationships. However, the crisis of opportunity concerned here is one of life service. "It is not a choice of the personality, based upon expedient or earthly motives, necessity or anything else. It is a choice based upon the relation of the soul to the personality."[12]

This is a two-phase process. Later we come to a 'crisis of expression' as to our use of Soul energy. Whereas other tests may have had a focus on one particular level, the crisis of expression occurs on all planes at once. It is part of the process by which our life of service can become clearly defined by the age of 49. We begin to know what we are about! Esoteric psychology suggests that initiation often occurs after the age of 50.

There is an important point reached around the age of 56 too.

> ... unless a certain measure of fusion [of Soul and personality] is established by the time fifty-six years of age is attained, it is seldom established later. After that age, a [person] may hold to the point achieved and foster [his/her] aspiration but the dynamic submergence of the personality in the will and life of the soul is rare after that time.[13]

This point of crisis leads into a period of seven years. How we respond to it will govern our life-direction — whether the Soul continues to use us as a vehicle of expression into old age, or whether there will be a gradual withdrawal. Where the Soul has taken hold of its personality mechanism to some degree, we will be increasingly engaged in service — the natural effect of Soul contact. Our identity may also be expanding in a way that transcends the individual self. The Soul is said to transcend separation. Sensitivity to the Soul brings us into a more inclusive and universal identity.

So throughout life there is constant movement with fresh Ray energy being drawn in. The Ray energies qualifying each vehicle help us to work out our own karma, and to meet the requirements in a particular life,

---

12. Alice A Bailey, *Discipleship in the New Age*, vol II (Lucis Press Ltd, London) p. 644.
13. Alice A Bailey, *Discipleship in the New Age*, vol I (Lucis Press Ltd, London) pp. 596–7.

ensuring balanced development of consciousness over a series of lives. The experience can be very much like swinging on a pendulum, over-developing one side of our nature, and then developing its opposite. It is an ongoing process in which the general movement is towards balance and mastery over the Ray energies with which we are brought into contact.

Rays governing specific stages

The seven Rays can have an over-arching influence over different stages of the individual life-cycle. The idea is that each of the Rays in sequence conditions or governs, to some degree, the stages of life. The first years might be conditioned by seventh Ray influence with its innate tendency to link spirit and matter. Could this energy play a major role in driving the spark of consciousness down into matter, into physical form and holding it there? The seventh Ray is very much connected to the physical plane, anchoring the Ray forces into form, allowing the subtle influences to find concrete expression in the material world. In those earliest years, following birth, the focus is largely on physical development and control.

For the subsequent period of latency, sixth Ray energy could be the major qualifying influence. The emphasis during this stage is on the appropriation of the emotional vehicle and there is a real affinity with the energies of the astral plane. It is a time when many children experience psychic phenomena, suggesting that they are open to astral contact. Children also learn to differentiate their personal feelings and to own them for themselves. Here, the sensitive or abused child will repress feelings too painful to be close to, burying them within their astral (emotional) nature, where they continue to exist and to affect that child, then and as an adult, until the knot of hurt is understood and released.

Such feelings may be held at bay during the stage of early adulthood, which sees the development of the thinking principle. This may be a connection to the influence of the fifth Ray of concrete thought. Mind becomes the focus of attention; this can often be at the expense of the feeling or desire nature. Feelings are denied, though they do not go away. Not everyone responds to the impulse of the fifth Ray; many will remain locked within their feeling natures, unable to achieve a measure of mental polarisation. Consciousness gets stuck, held back by an absorption in the thrill of feeling and emotion, or astral psychic contact.

The crisis of mid-life is the period in which opposite tendencies meet, in which past experiences and future expectations conspire together, often stimulating inner conflict. Is this not a period characterised for many as a struggle to find greater harmony, to learn to work with the inner nature and to find ways of expressing themselves that harmonise with the way they are? We might also think not only of the tendency of the fourth Ray to establish harmony through conflict but also how this energy is on what is called the 2-4-6 Ray line. It is the feeling line and it may be that its influence during mid-life also allows earlier feelings to bubble to the surface once more. Yet repressed and suppressed feelings may not emerge to confront the mental focus achieved during adult life. Can a more whole person emerge? Can harmony be found? Can some measure of personal integration be achieved?

With this hypothesis we would expect to see third Ray energy of active intelligence qualifying the individual life-expression following the mid-life period. Perhaps the scope for truly intelligent activity is most likely at this time for those who have negotiated mid-life and established within them a tendency towards greater wholeness. From their integrated state and with increasing responsiveness to the Soul nature, they can carry their life forward with intelligence.

The third Ray is linked to the plane of the higher mind. If mid-life has seen the achievement of some measure of Soul contact, the potential is there in that life to extend the individual thought-life to the higher levels of the mental plane. This is facilitated by third Ray influence at this time. It is as if the fruits of past experience and development are synthesised; Ray qualities that have become 'fixed' within the individual are in some way blended with the third Ray quality now seeking greater expression, to be carried into the next stage of life.

As we move towards late life, love-wisdom, the energy of the second Ray, provides a major stimulus. Who do we see as the wise ones? Those who have experienced life, who have worked through the earlier stages and gained knowledge and understanding, and whose consciousness has moved on through the different stages of growth. They will have had much to assimilate and to synthesise into the second Ray at this stage. Those who have much to bring into the process at this time of life will blend their intelligence and knowledge with love and guide others by their wisdom. They will have understood their experiences in the light of the Soul. They will provide others with light on their paths through words of wisdom and acts of compassion.

Is it not a great tragedy of western life that there is little respect from the young for the elderly? A bridge across the generations is desperately needed; a blending of youthful idealism with the wisdom of experience. It should be possible to bring them closer, especially if there is a common energy line linking young people (sixth Ray) with those responding to the second Ray impulse at this stage of later life (Figure 6). This energy line offers a clear opportunity.

The final stage of life, which leads up to death, can be seen to be largely shaped by the energy of Will. Is this not the goal of a full life, to align with Will? Not everyone reaches this. We all find our natural level and carry that energy into the rest of our lives, but for those who arrive at this period with the capacity to respond to Will, it is truly a life of fulfilment. What is it that finally breaks the connection and allows the individual consciousness to pass through the transition which the world calls death but which the wise know as entrance into 'life more abundant'? The energy of Will.

Figure 6 shows how, following mid-life, we may carry the energy of the Rays of Aspect into expression through our personality natures. It also indicates why people in the third Ray stage may have an affinity with those at the fifth Ray stage of life; and the same regarding second and sixth Ray stages and first and seventh Ray stages. We might also see it as indicating that Soul energy is being carried down into expression during this latter phase of life, assuming Soul contact has been established and maintained.

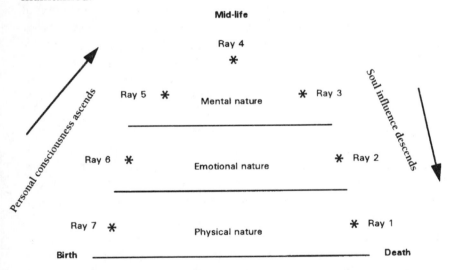

Figure 6. Life-cycle with achieved Soul contact by mid-life

There is another facet of this to consider, for, whilst Soul energy is brought into the world, consciousness may continue to expand into Soul realms and beyond. As a result, a living link in consciousness develops, spanning the world of the personality and that of the Soul. Figure 7 represents this.

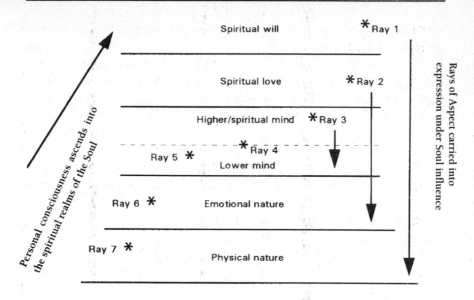

Figure 7. Consciousness reaches into spiritual realms

Here we see the possibility of a conscious link being created within the individual, spanning spiritual and temporal realms. It may be that in one life the link is established with the higher mind and that it will require further lifetimes of experience and conscious growth for the individual to open to the next realm of the Soul, that of spiritual love. Once again we come back to the idea that each life is to a certain point a recapitulation of what has gone before. We hopefully move through life to a critical point from which we are then ready to break new ground. Hence life can be a voyage of rediscovery.

The idea that we can generate a thread of conscious connections with spiritual realms is a powerful one and, in the context of Life as a process through many lives, can begin to indicate a purpose and a direction. Maybe evolution is about building a bridge in consciousness spanning the material and the spiritual worlds. Perhaps it is the conscious application of spiritual energy and impulse that is our role and reason for existing, resulting in some form of redemption or purification of substance in the earthly realm.

Where Soul contact has not been made

Like all that has been considered in this chapter, the idea of the Rays governing periods in the life-cycle in sequence is a model to help us understand what happens and why we may experience and act as we do at different stages. This outline of Ray influence on the life-cycle assumes progressive development for the individual, leading to some measure of spiritual awareness. What of those who have not yet reached this stage? Do they also come under the influence of the Ray energies in their sequence? Perhaps, yet in a way that stimulates not spiritual development so much as a personal focus. If there is not an expansion of consciousness towards the Soul nature, perhaps the Ray energies manifest more fully in their lower, self-centred form of expression.

Consider, for instance, the latter half of life. The third Ray might be seen as manipulative, devious and selfish in its expression. It may not stimulate a raising of thought to the plane of the higher mind, but rather stimulate any crystallising tendency that has begun within the individual thought-life. Indeed, this may then be the basis for a crystallising process throughout the personality in line with the ancient axiom of "energy follows thought".

The second Ray energy as it influences later life might be distorted into greater self-love or even self-pity, particularly if despair obscures any measure of experienced ego-integrity. It may also be directed towards a love of the past or towards the expression of sentimentality. It would encourage a phase in which love energy, which could have been expansive, turns inwards, and love of self and the things that have made the person what they are become the focus for that love. It can become a very material and possessive force.

The final stage may then see a powerful self-will manifesting. This may be positive in the sense that it drives the individual on in a constant and at times desperate struggle to retain physical life. It may turn in on the individual, driving them towards an even greater self-centred focus and the emergence of a self-will that is fiercely, and unrealistically, independent, before the final release.

It might be helpful to think of it in terms of spirals. The individual spirals out from birth on their journey through life. If they achieve Soul contact and can make this the centre of their lives then the spiral moves away from being centred on the personal self and begins to spiral around the Soul. This represents an expansion of consciousness. However, if this movement is not achieved, the spiral movement contracts and consciousness remains centred around the personality.

We do, however, need to guard against being too precise or judgemental with these ideas. It may not be this simple. The extreme expressions may well occur, but there is going to be a good mixture of Ray expression within each individual, some positive and Soul-qualified, some conditioned by personality reactions of a separative nature. Only an achieved state of perfection can hope to provide a vehicle for carrying Ray energy into its fullest and most positive expression. Few are perfect. We all colour Ray impulse by our imperfections.

What happens when a life is cut short?

Many spiritual traditions suggest that generally speaking there is an underlying plan for each life. Whether it is fulfilled will depend on the choices made by the individual and how they handle the situations that they attract in their lives. In cases of accident or disaster in which the individual life is shortened in a way that cuts through the life-cycle, certain stages will not have been experienced, and perhaps may be extended in a future life as compensation. Or it may generate some form of trauma, and a process of compensation occurs after death.

When a life has a kind of natural shortness, when a biological process has brought about the death of the form, perhaps the stages are more concentrated rather than some simply not taking place. Maybe the shortness of the life is the result of choices made and attitudes held, or is a learning process both for the individual concerned and those who are close to them.

Time and timing

It seems reasonable that through a natural life, whether long or short, each energy phase will occur. Certain stages may be lengthened or shortened to promote balance or growth, or even to take advantage of the availability of energies from other sources. It also seems reasonable to avoid setting definite time periods for these Ray influences. Their cyclic flow has to be seen in relation to consciousness and not to the time-bound form. We are, however, very time-dominated in our thinking about life processes, indeed about most things. For the Soul, I feel, time as we know it does not exist. So lengths of time may be of less significance. Of more importance are the energies involved, how they are applied and when they are applied. Timing, rather than time, may be more significant.

It can be helpful to think about time less as a linear experience and more as a cyclic flow. The time that we create in our minds is divided up, a kind of bit-by-bit experience. We talk of moments of time and measure them in seconds or minutes. Yet subjectively we all know that some minutes last longer than others, some hours pass speedily whilst others go on for ever. Some will live more in 20 years than others in 80, or in their last ten years than in the rest of their life put together.

The more we live our lives 'to time' the more we actually divert our attention from experiencing the present to the full. We may use perceived lack of time as an excuse not to do things. Maybe we should carry the idea that time will flow around what we need to do, rather than constrain our efforts. We know that when a real crisis occurs our experience of time can slow down and we achieve far more in a short space of time. Time is elastic and consciousness in some mysterious way allows us to stretch it. Perhaps each life-cycle is elastic-time and it is in our hands, hearts and minds as to whether we will stretch or contract it.

Conclusion

With Ray energies governing particular stages in life, and individual vehicles also governed by Ray energy, care must be taken when seeking an understanding of psychological development. To appreciate the subtlety of this view of psychology does not call on the intellect as much as it does on the intuition. There is a role for reason *and* for feeling. To discriminate between the subtle energies that shape us requires great sensitivity. It also requires us to be sensitive to a more universal perspective towards our lives. The life-cycle may be broken down into stages, but in truth it can only be understood when seen as a whole, and in its context of a series of lives.

For the individual who seeks deeper understanding and self-knowledge, there is only one psychological reality — *the here and now*. As we learn to know ourselves more fully in the present moment, whatever stage of life we may be at, we open doors and touch the unrealised possibilities that are the seeds of our psychological future. An appreciation of the role of Ray energy will help us to understand what may be taking place in our psychological development, and what unrealised potential exists, seeking expression in and through our lives and relationships.

Colouring Psychological Growth

What is colour? To our physical eyes colour is the visible effect of the differentiation of white light into frequency bands. Colour is a form of vibration. It enables us to discriminate within the visible, electromagnetic spectrum. Although visible colour is only a small range of vibration, its sevenfold nature provides a correspondence to the sevenfold nature of creation and the Seven Rays. We know that there is a realm of the invisible within the electromagnetic spectrum measured by scientific instrumentation, which can show us where fields of energies exist and overlap. So often the electrical impulses are translated into colour for us to see on computer screens. Some people, who are sensitive, claim to be able to see subtle energies either through the physical eye (etheric vision) or clairvoyantly (the astral plane).

Perception

Our own bodies are composed of energy — physical/etheric, emotional, mental and spiritual. They are bodies of colour. Through a sensitivity to colour we can learn a great deal about ourselves, for colours associated with energy states can directly affect our perception. Let us take the scenario of someone becoming angry whilst driving — they might literally 'see red' and an offending vehicle might appear that colour, whilst, if the driver had calmed down, he might have seen it in a totally different 'light' as blue or green or whatever. Maybe the person had so much anger in themselves that they had generated red within their own energy field and through this, like a coloured lens, perceived red on the object of their anger.

If we have sensitivity to subtle energies, when we perceive colour we need to realise that we are looking through the colours of our own energy fields. Also, the impacts reaching us from outside will be coloured by our own vibrations. So one person may bring feelings into a relationship which, when they touch us, energise feelings within us that we then sense, but which may not be the same as those of the other person. Our own feeling content may be stimulated into our conscious awareness to 'colour' our perception of what the other person is experiencing.

It could also be that we enter into an intense emotional state and memories of similar feelings bring images to consciousness that 'colour' our perception of the present. We become so full of these feelings or 'colours' from the past that we do not see or feel clearly or realistically.

Another facet of perception is whether we actually see the same things. Is the red that I perceive the same as the red that you perceive? Can we ever know if my green is your green? We assume that we all experience the same colours, but do we? Maybe the wavelength of light entering my eye triggers a different experience in my brain from that in yours. We might then take this further and ask whether colour actually exists? Or is it simply our way of perceiving and differentiating objects in the same way that our computers differentiate energy fields and produce coloured images on a screen? There are deep mysteries in relation to colour and I feel our current knowledge has only touched the surface. Indeed, that is what colour is in our form world, evidence of a surface. It does not tell us what lies beneath, but might it hint at hidden depths?

Colour healing

This is a vast subject. There is the exoteric application of colour where healing is required on the physical/etheric levels. Then there is the more esoteric form of healing in which colour is used to stimulate the healing process on mental and emotional levels. Here, however, I want to explore a more psychological approach to healing and colour, using colour more as a metaphor or a language to help us think about how human energy fields might affect each other when brought into relationship. Yet we know that in reality colour is more, much more, than metaphor. The presence of physical colour can affect mood and awaken memories or generate feelings. It can heal and it can disorientate as well.

I remember a visit to Savill Gardens, in Surrey, England a couple of years back. It was Spring. The azaleas and rhododendrons were at their best — incredibly clear, bright colours: pinks, whites, reds, yellows, purples, seemingly every colour and shade you could imagine, and more. Walking along a footpath with large azalea bushes on either side I experienced what I can only describe as the feeling of being painted. It was a remarkable sensation. I felt renewed, refreshed, revitalised and it seemed to be to do with the colours that were so close to me on either side. Whilst there is colour in energy, there is certainly energy in colour! Lynn described my expression in terms of looking 'blissed-out' with a huge grin across my face. I was not aware of that, I simply knew that it felt good. Yet as I entered that path I had no expectation, I was not trying to generate an experience, it simply arose as I walked through the colours.

Colour and the Seven Rays

It is widely acknowledged that *all is energy* as Einstein showed. Earlier we looked at the differentiation of the One Light into seven streams of energy — the Seven Rays — which we each embody in various permutations within our own energy fields. We are also sensitive to them as they radiate from other sources — people, kingdoms in nature, planets or the great zodiacal constellations. We exist within an extremely complex interweaving of Ray energy, each having its own distinctive colour which changes in relation to the density or subtlety of the substance through which it flows.

An energy stream flowing into the human energy fields, touching different levels of vibration, may change the colour, the energy's 'appearance'. It might take the form of one colour within one aspect of your nature, and another colour elsewhere.

Human relationships

In any human interaction there is an exchange of energy. Sometimes this can be a very magnetic exchange; for instance, between partners or between a group of co-workers who are co-operating on a project. However, the energies do not always interact well and friction can ensue. Could it be that, using the language of colour, there is no blending but rather a clash?

When two people meet, a very definite energy interaction occurs. Energy can flow powerfully in either direction, in much the same way as an electric current is induced by a potential difference. It may take some while for this exchange to reach a point of free flow, or balance. The bond of trust takes time to develop. It requires each to bring themselves fully into the encounter. Energies/colours are mixing. New shades may appear, stimulating new forms of expression or interest. Sensitivities previously not realised may emerge. The tone of a person's life may begin to change. An important part of what we might term 'esoteric counselling' lies in establishing a quality of relationship with the client that resonates to the Soul. This has certain similarities to transpersonal psychology.

Esoteric psychology suggests that perfection draws imperfection to the surface. The Soul is perfect. When resonance to the Soul is achieved in the therapeutic relationship, or indeed in any human relationship, the blocks and hindrances to growth and to coping with life are drawn powerfully to the surface to be faced and worked through. The Soul is also

naturally 'group conscious'. This may be why group work can be powerfully therapeutic — the supportive group relationship having a greater
capacity for focusing Soul quality. The group holds the capacity for a
greater range and intensity of colour within its dynamic energy field.

We express Ray energy through our individual personalities. The Soul
has a particular Ray energy. The quality and type of energy to which a
person resonates is brought into the therapeutic relationship. One implication may be that, for people with certain difficulties, healing will be
most likely when the interaction is with a person of a particular Ray type.
This Ray energy may 'colour' the client in such a way as to offset imbalance and stimulate healing. In some instances, similar Ray influences
working through the client and therapist may be most beneficial. In others it may require the introduction of a different Ray.

This is not to suggest the presence of some magic wand to be waved
from Soul levels to make imperfections vanish in an instant. The blocks,
hindrances and traumas that limit growth towards 'whole-being' need to
be resolved. This can take time and be extremely painful. It can also foster a sense of joy, vitality and liberation. There are many approaches to
resolving blocks, many psychological models to explain the processes
that can help to move us on. These include: integrating conscious/un-
conscious content; realigning with the actualising tendency; and creating
a new script for living. Individuals have to find a way to achieve greater
psychological wholeness that is right for them.

Of course, Ray energy can stimulate both wholesome and not so
wholesome expression. For instance, third Ray energy stimulates clarity
of intellect, patience and the great quality of adaptability. Yet it can also
stimulate selfish manipulation, intense materialism and criticism. The
outcome largely depends on the focus of consciousness. This leads us
into the topic of 'glamour'. The Ray of Love-Wisdom can stimulate
glamours of the love of being loved and of fear based upon undue sensitivity. The Ray of Idealism and Devotion can encourage glamours of
sentimentality and fanaticism.

Glamour

Glamour is an esoteric, technical term. It refers to the effect when our
desire or feeling nature distorts experiences and perceptions. When we
are centred in our personal feelings and something touches them in a
powerful way, they vibrate very easily. We can experience an overwhelming sense of emotional reaction that may be quite out of proportion to
the initial contact. The emotions can feel like a very wobbly jelly. Once it

starts shaking it takes time to settle down again.

People whose consciousness is centred in their feeling nature thrive on the thrill of emotional vibration. Things take on importance that in reality are of little significance, but they *feel* so momentous. We use the word glamorous in a positive sense in our culture — the rich and the fashionable — who we are encouraged to admire for their lifestyle. The glossy magazines are full of images to entice our feeling natures to vibrate. Quantity of lifestyle is presented as quality. Yet from the angle of the Soul the glamours and the glamorous are of little moment. It is the quality of the human heart and mind that really matters.

Each Ray has its own set of glamours which are essentially limited and distorted expressions of that energy. As you can imagine, the first Ray can stimulate a glamour of power as the be all and end all of life; the second Ray, a glamour of love in a personal sense; and the third Ray, a glamour of activity as being what life is really all about. The fourth Ray might express itself through a glamour of struggle and conflict, or of preserving harmony at all costs; the fifth Ray would glamorise thought and intellect above all else. The sixth Ray would express itself through a glamour along the lines of, "if it feels right to me, then it *must* be right" which, in extreme form, can lead to fanaticism. Personal feelings are not always right at all! The seventh Ray would see order and organisation as the answer to everything. What energy do you think lies behind the constant urge of companies to restructure at huge expense, only to then undergo another similar process a few months later because it has not worked out?

This has to be a simplification but it conveys a sense of the effects of glamour in relation to the Rays. We are each complex mixes of Ray energy so we may carry a real mixture of glamour within our nature. How can we dispel it so that we can see ourselves and others with truth and clarity? First of all we have to recognise its presence, and the mind comes into play as we seek to step back from the emotional reactions in which glamour is rooted. A mind sensitive to the light of the Soul will see through it. We then have to substitute behaviours that stem from glamour with those that are reasonable to the enlightened mind.

A therapist with a different Ray energy may enable the client to see around their glamour. Or maybe the therapist has worked through that glamour and subjectively radiates a light of understanding into the therapeutic relationship which enables the client to see beyond it. The aim is to allow energy to colour the client through the quality of presence that has been established in the relationship. A free-flowing energy exchange takes place. In the language of colour, new shades, tints and blends which indicate Soul influence will appear as energies of a purer vibration, tones which have become available for assimilation and absorption.

However, if the therapist has not resolved a glamour, it will be introduced into the relationship and, if it resonates with that of the client, will produce problems for them both. The classic example is second Ray glamour inducing overwhelming feelings of love between client and therapist. It is easy to stand back and say that it should not happen, but it does and it is a powerful experience from which to break free. One reason why it is so common may be that many therapists themselves embody second Ray energy with its healing and caring quality.

In the final analysis, total healing involves the drawing into expression of the client's own Soul. In certain circumstances this may require them to work with someone having similar Ray energies. At other times, a person with a different set of energies may provide greater therapeutic potential.

Meditations may be used to invoke particular Ray energies. However, this requires intuitive development in the person assigning the meditation or creative visualisations. Seeing psychological growth in the light of the Seven Rays opens up fresh possibilities both for working and for understanding the therapeutic process. I hope that, as human consciousness fuses more completely with the Soul, and the science of the Seven Rays is firmly established as a topic for study, investigation and application, this will become an accepted technique and an established part of psychological training and therapy.

Shaping the Nations of the World

The Seven Ray model suggests that the whole of creation is the effect of the interweaving of seven basic energies:

Ray One   The Ray of Will or Power
Ray Two   The Ray of Love-Wisdom
Ray Three The Ray of Active Intelligence and Adaptability
Ray Four   The Ray of Harmony through Conflict, of Beauty and Art
Ray Five   The Ray of Concrete Knowledge and of Science
Ray Six   The Ray of Idealism and Devotion
Ray Seven The Ray of Ceremonial Order and Ritual

The world's nationalities are governed by Ray energy, in a similar fashion to the individual. Each has a Soul Ray and a personality Ray. The major cities, in particular the capitals, are also conditioned by Soul and personality Ray influences. This may sound rather strange at first reading. How can a city or a nation be governed by energies that also in some way condition human personality types? We come back to the basic premise that creation has a sevenfold quality — and this means *all* of creation, everything that has existence is subject to the influence of Ray energy.

Once we grasp the enormity of the idea that everything is subject to similar influences, although the response that these bring forth may differ widely, we have a common thread from which to build our understanding of the world and the forms of life that exist in it. I am reminded of perception tests involving complex patterns that conceal a letter or a number which, when seen in a certain way, reveal their secret. Looking at the world, at the many styles of human living, we can sometimes find it hard to recognise similarities and patterns amidst the complexity and diversity. Yet they are there and the Seven Ray model can enable us to cast a light on our experiences that helps us to identify the common qualities finding expression.

Understanding which Rays govern a given nation gives insight into why its people have particular characteristics. We can begin to see why nation states interact with each other in the way that they do. This is quite a leap from personal psychology, but in the final analysis it is the people that make up a city or a nation, not the geography. It is the bringing together of consciousness in relationship that creates community. So we should not be surprised that communities (local, national or international) are subject to the same influences as the individuals of which they are composed.

Let us look at the Ray energies of some nations:[14]

Nation	Soul Ray	Personality Ray
Austria	Fourth	Fifth
Brazil	Fourth	Second
Britain	Second	First
China	First	Third
France	Fifth	Third
Germany	Fourth	First
India	First	Fourth
Italy	Sixth	Fourth
Russia	Seventh	Sixth
Spain	Sixth	Seventh
USA	Second	Sixth

14.   Alice A Bailey, *The Destiny of the Nations* (The Lucis Press Ltd, London) p. 67.

From this tabulation we can see some interesting relationships between nations. We will not explore them all, but introduce some of the Ray qualities as they find expression, to give an introduction to a Seven Rays view of national attitudes and potential.

Britain

Some countries seem to have natural affinities with each other, others not. Britain and the USA have the same Soul Rays — the Ray of Love-Wisdom. Yet their personality rays are quite different. Britain's first Ray personality revealed itself through the power of empire and in being an historical centre for the evolution of government. In the days of empire the power Ray as an expression of her expansive second Ray drove her influence across the world.

Today, Britain's challenge lies in learning to wield her powerful personality in service to the whole of her people and, on a greater sweep of the spiral of life, to humanity as a whole. For this she needs the inclusive note of her second Ray Soul. The first Ray has helped Britain to be a visible and vocal player in the world, she now has to choose for whom she wishes to use her voice: national self-interest or the wider needs of humanity and the planet.

It is possible that Britain's first Ray energy (finding strong political and governmental expression) is drawing her closer to Europe, however much she distrusts that which she cannot control and dominate herself. Is it a truism that we react against the traits in others that are in us too? Britain seems to react against the threats of European domination and bureaucracy! She struggles to stand with resolute determination for her own interests.

USA

The USA has a powerful sixth Ray personality. This energy, linked as we have seen to the emotional plane and the adolescent stage of life, has a certain exuberant quality about it. It can also stimulate an urge towards militarism as well as devotion and idealism in general. Where is the USA directing this energy? It tends towards material well-being and the American dream. Is this a dream also focused on encouraging planetary and human well-being?

Sixth Ray energy can encourage a tendency towards a rather 'knee-jerk' reaction to events, making it difficult for a coherent and thoughtful response to take place. It can stimulate an urge to rush in without due preparation for what will follow. Wisdom is rarely reactive. Yet it is not procrastinating either.

The note of the second Ray emanates from the Soul of the USA, urging her to expand her focus and lift and universalise her ideals towards human unity, co-operation and sharing. Like Britain, she has tremendous energy potential to serve the whole and to take the lead in fostering a 'culture of caring' that is so desperately needed in our world.

The great ideal of freedom is held up as it rightly should be. Yet freedom has many faces. Freedom to be and to grow out of our inner resources of human potential, or to grow outwardly through economic exploitation? Freedom, if it is to be expressive of the human Soul, is linked with responsibility for the effects of our actions, whether we like it or not. In our world of economic and ecological interconnectedness there is no escaping responsibility for our actions. Our individual choices affect others around the world; our collective choices have even greater effect. For America, with her power and potential to lead humanity forward, crucial choices lie ahead. Humanity needs an idealistic lead towards greater love and wisdom in all areas of her collective expression. The USA has the energy potential to provide this lead.

Russia

Turning next to Russia, we see again a connection between two countries, this time through the energy of the sixth Ray. The USA and Russia are, in their own style and emphasis, equally intensely idealistic. Both have revealed a militaristic face to the world and an urge to impose their ideals on everyone else. Can they now work together, to evolve a common ideal, to work towards drawing on their Soul impulses to hold the ideal of a new order qualified by love-wisdom? There is a very real opportunity for the Russian people in response to the note of their seventh Ray Soul, to carve out a new order in their country, if materialistic idealism does not distort it and place power back into the hands of a spirit of separateness.

Russia seems to embody the collective human dilemma as she seeks to move from a dominant sixth Ray influence towards a sensitivity to the note of the seventh Ray. Her struggles are humanity's struggle. She is grappling with the urge to find a new ideal, caught between the casting out of the old, totalitarian regime and pressure to embrace the western model of economic development. What a choice! Can her idealism, however, be reoriented towards a new order based on the principles of unity, sharing and solidarity? It may seem hard to imagine during this difficult transition phase and yet great forces are at work and we cannot yet know to what final goal they may be urging the Russian people. Transition always involves breakdown and confusion before recreation and rebirth. What is important is that the nations of the world harness their strengths and potential and learn to recognise the glamours that distort their expression and natural emphasis.

France

France's Ray energies are quite different. They reveal themselves through her scientific nature. However, the fifth Ray can also be very isolating in its expression and foster a great deal of self-centredness. Her challenge it seems lies in bringing her scientific thought into intelligent expression for the common good of humanity. Her brilliant mind can be opened to the light of the Soul (she has the energy potential for this) and directed towards revealing that which is for the good of the whole. If she can achieve this she will bring much-needed illumination both into European thought and the mind of humanity. However, for this to occur she will need to negate her tendencies towards self-interest and manipulation.

She has little to connect her to the USA and Britain in terms of her Soul and personality Rays. This can be a problem when co-operation and communication are vital, for instance, in trade agreements. Negotiations between Europe and the USA on this matter in the 1990s have highlighted these differences and, while Britain and France might agree on some areas of European interest that coincide with their own perceived national interest, there remains an unease in their relationship within the European trading framework.

Germany

Staying in Europe, Germany may reveal more of its Soul nature now that it has re-unified, although a great deal of adjustment is obviously required. At least her personality is no longer split and her energy fragmented. Her Soul Ray of harmony through conflict certainly reveals much about her history and her present internal difficulties. Powerful forces are at work and she really does have a tough time coping with her energies and finding a way to give them wholesome expression.

The fourth Ray is expected to become a more potent influence in the next century and so we may see a stimulation of Germany's Soul expression. Perhaps then her rich heritage of philosophical thought and musical composition will once again emerge into prominence. She has the potential to become a major centre of culture at the heart of Europe, and with Britain (through their common first Ray) a focus for power used inclusively and harmoniously.

Her challenge lies in preserving balance and allowing this to qualify her strong first Ray personality. We have seen in the past her struggle to achieve this and how the power Ray can sweep into expression seeking to impose extreme regimes on the people — and on the world.

Italy

Beauty and art are qualities we naturally associate with Italy. Her intense idealism and devotion (sixth Ray) can be directed towards religion, fashion, Ferraris and all things Italian. Earlier this century her idealism turned towards fascism (as did Spain's who also has sixth Ray energy in her Soul). The Italians are a passionate people, you only have to think of their devotion to football. They are also a colourful people with a flair for design and elegance in the search for harmony and beauty in form (fourth Ray).

Like some other European countries, Italy is in a certain sense a young nation borne out of the gathering of fiercely independent city states and principalities. Politically she is in constant conflict, never able to hold down a consistent and steady approach. Italian politics is certainly colourful and volatile, a good example of fourth and sixth Ray influence. Can she help shape and give colour to the new ideals that are required for life in the 21st century? She has the energy potential for this, but she must be prepared to think in global terms and establish harmony within her own political and economic life. Perhaps as much as anything she can offer the evocative power of beauty to the world through her creativity in form.

Brazil

Brazil is also governed by fourth Ray energy (Soul) along with the second Ray (personality). It is an interesting combination, particularly as the zodiacal rulers of her Soul (Leo) and personality (Virgo) convey the same energies through their ruling planets. There is a suggestion that when a nation is governed by the second and the fourth Rays it will prove to have a significant role in determining human destiny.

This idea reminds me of the UNCED gathering (Earth Summit) in Brazil in 1992. Was this not a crucial opportunity for humanity to create new values for living and to nurture the ideal of ecological sustainability? It certainly established sustainability as the partner to development. It inspired the creation of many new initiatives and networks around the planet, encouraging communication and co-operation on a scale previously unseen. Whilst the outer activity is vital and heartening (although the scope for far greater sensitivity to the ecology of the Earth remains all too apparent) we need also to think of the ideas and the ideals that emerged from UNCED, and the process of consultation that has developed to ensure that they are not lost. The second Ray is a building energy and without doubt the Earth Summit offered a foundation on which we could build a sustainable future.

China

Finally, let us consider China. She has some challenging energies to work with too: a first Ray Soul and a third Ray personality. Third Ray energy can find expression through a practical view of life. The Chinese people do exhibit a practical attitude, one example being the way they have sought to establish an internal system for feeding their vast population. Yet this same energy can lead to webs of deceit and manipulation, a separative expression of this powerful energy.

China's struggle seems to be concerned with bringing power and will into right relationship with creativity and economic interplay. Without doubt, she will be a powerful economy in the next century. Her development, if she follows the western model, has to have a severe environmental impact. Whether China uses her natural will energy to serve her own material needs, or whether a wider vision will dominate has yet to be seen. Maybe she will offer humanity a fresh vision of economic interplay, demonstrating how people's needs can be met in a sustainable way. Whatever she decides, she will be a force to be reckoned with on the world stage.

Conclusion

This is a rather brief introduction to how we can see the nations in the light of Ray energy. *Destiny of the Nations* by Alice Bailey goes more deeply into this topic. What is important when exploring the application of Ray energy in human life is that we should avoid being dogmatic. We are trying to make sense of complex interactions which may not have a final definitive explanation that the human mind can grasp. We each have to

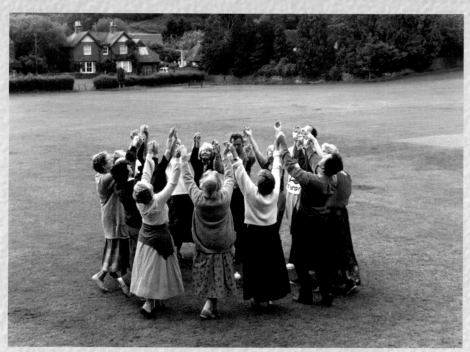

Dancing Kore at Brook, Surrey

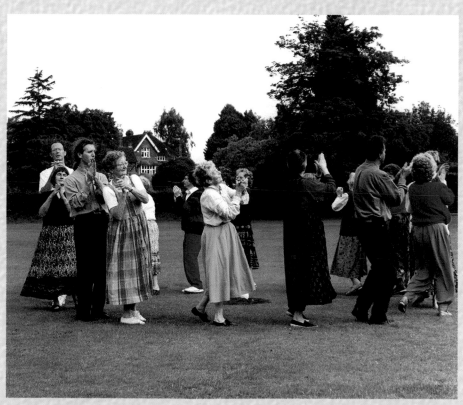

Dancing Nigun Atik at Brook, Surrey

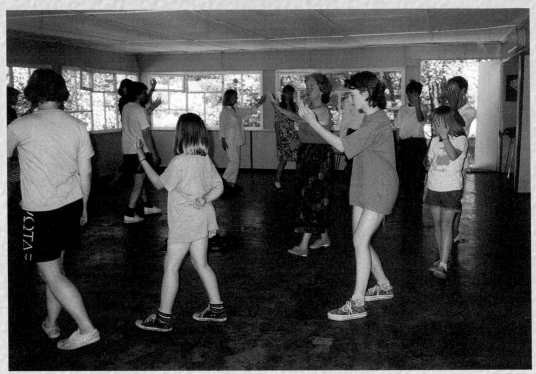

Learning Samiotissa in Poland, 1995

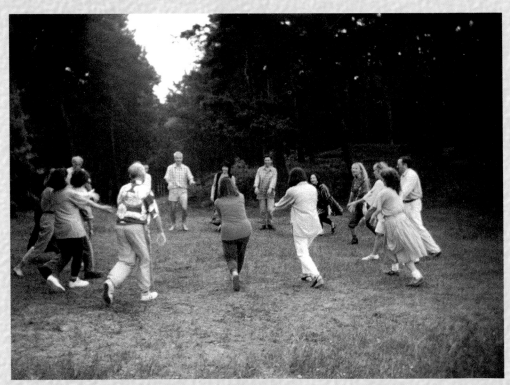

Dancing Od lo ahavti dai in Poland, 1996

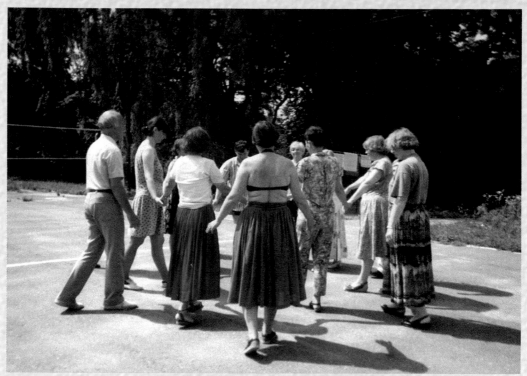

Dancing the Dance of Unity in Poland, 1997

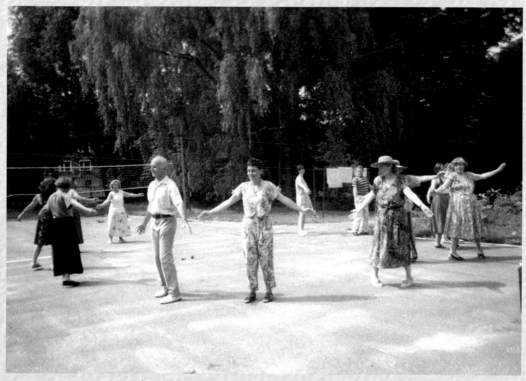

Dancing Santo in Poland, 1997

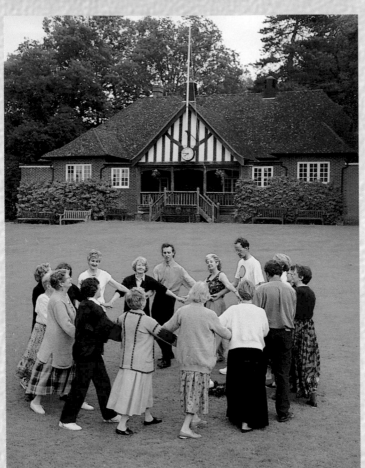

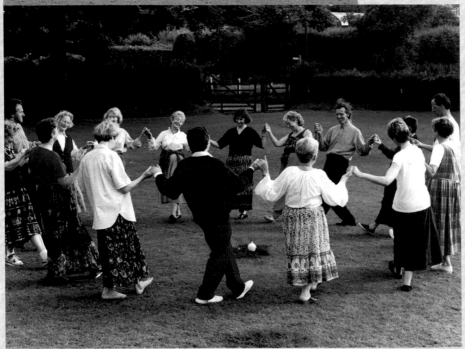

Dancing Kangaleftes at Brook, Surrey

try to understand what occurs for ourselves and, as we gain insight, maybe we can learn to co-operate with the vast forces and energies that are shaping human destiny.

Without doubt, the idea that nations are governed by powerful energies which have their own essential qualities opens up a whole new perspective on international relations and the art of diplomacy. Perhaps in the future nations will work together in ways that honour each other's energy potential and complement each other's natural qualities, rather than the current world order which seems to involve co-operation only when it coincides with national self-interest. There is a planetary and a human interest at stake too, and this is surely more important in the final analysis than the preservation of artificial borders and political and economic blocs.

I envisage that tomorrow's world will see a transcendence of the nation state as we know it. Today we are just beginning to step out towards a world that will no longer hold in highest esteem national self-interest. The realisation will surely pervade all hearts and minds that individual interest lies with that which is for the common good, whether we talk of the individual human being, community or nation state. Do you think this is far-fetched? How much of today's world dwelt only in the realm of the unthinkable 50 years ago? Who dares to predict the face of the world in 50 or 100 years' time with any certainty?

Now is a time for radical thought based on sound principles, for vision that encompasses all that is good and creative within the human being. As the strategic thinkers tell us, forget the obstacles, get a vision of where you want to be, then find the realistic path that will take you there, and start walking along that path. We need people of vision who can think beyond the length of a parliament or term of office. We need the human will (not just the political will, because it is not simply the responsibility of politicians) to drive us on. We need a vision to live and work towards a world that will provide for human need, and respect ecological balance. The Rays foster diversity of expression and an enriching experience for us all. Can we unite in our common humanity and our common spiritual essence to allow diversity to flourish in such a way that it is not distorted by separative and selfish attitudes? Can we afford any other vision?

Call to Love

From those early days of thirsting after spiritual and esoteric knowledge, through a phase of consolidation as I built on this knowledge through my work at the Lucis Trust, and then a movement on to seek out my own insight and knowledge from within myself, I feel as though I have followed a natural progression. I began with an inner sense of a need for something. I desperately sought it out, generally looking outside myself as this is how education usually encourages us to find answers to questions (whilst the true meaning of *educare*, the root of our word education, is 'to lead out' from within our own nature).

Having found teachings and ideas that I could relate to and which fitted well with my own developing world-view, I found myself struggling to live those ideas in my work and daily life. Sometimes succeeding, often falling flat on my face and only in hindsight realising I had got it wrong again! Then endeavouring to turn it all into a learning experience. How easy it is to write that our disasters are really learning experiences! It is kind of comforting. It can also shield us from really taking a long, hard and honest look at ourselves and our creations, allowing us to avoid taking responsibility, particularly when we seem to constantly pass from self-induced disaster to self-induced disaster, creating lots of learning experiences for ourselves of course, and lots of pain and confusion in those around us.

In the final analysis we have all got to find ways that enable us to know ourselves. We have to know who we are, why we function the way we do and, taking a firm grip on our often unruly and separative nature, drive it in the direction that we honestly and truly want to travel in.

Only the Soul can hold the reins, not the bellicose and inflated personality that is so proud of its little and usually transient achievement in our material world. There is a story in *The Labours of Hercules*[15] in which Hercules has to capture wild horses that are devastating the countryside. Hercules, expressing the power of the Soul, achieves his goal, but on his return journey he leaves his friend Abderis to control them and bring them along. They turn on Abderis and rend him to shreds. Hercules has walked on ahead feeling his own importance and glorying in his achievement. But Abderis lay dead.

The story illustrates how difficult it is to control our lower natures. When we slip back into being the self-important personality, glorying in our achievement, we are lining ourselves up for a fall.

---

15.   Alice A Bailey *The Labours of Hercules* (The Lucis Press Ltd, London).

On my journey of personal growth, if I have learned anything, it is this — the Soul, the spiritual Self, is my Reality. All else is a field of experience that can be transformed into a field of service through the presence of the Soul. Growth is for me about the struggle to rediscover my identity as the spiritual Self, so that I may then truly live to some greater purpose free of the limitation of a sense of separateness.

We can no longer afford to allow our creative expression to be dominated by petty personalities and greed. We have billions of people to feed, billions of people to house and to clothe, billions of people that, like us, would like to live with dignity.

My experience of visiting Israel has consolidated my belief in the importance of having some form of personal contact with people in other countries. I remain convinced that we respond differently to news, particularly bad news, when we have a personal contact in a trouble-spot. I know how easy it is to experience what has been glibly called 'compassion fatigue', but can 'compassion fatigue' exist for us when we know someone living in a place where painful events are occurring? Our sense of humanity will not allow it.

Yes, it hurts us to see some of the scenes that we do on our television, or to read reports and see pictures in our newspapers — and these are only the ones that we are allowed to see, the really sharp images never reach us. Yet it seems to me that we need to hurt inside. We need to feel the pain of others. We need to stand in solidarity with those who suffer daily. This is my struggle as a counsellor and therapist, but I know that it helps.

I ask myself, "how can they feel my love if I cannot feel their pain?" This seems to really sum it up for me, somehow. Think about it. It is all very well thinking light and love and believing that this is going to change everything. This is good and positive to do. It contributes, but alone it is not enough. We need human-to-human, person-to-person connections if our hearts are truly to be effective in allowing a flow of love to occur. We have to engage with people, touch them and be touched by them. We must see their woe and then, in communion with them, let the light and love of the Soul blaze forth. Do not just imagine it, *live it, be it, make it real*. Spiritual knowledge always brings responsibility to live it within our own circle of expression and relationship. The world is today that circle.

It is hard and it is painful. It is easy to feel dragged down by what we witness in our troubled world. Yet we cannot look the other way. We have to be hurt too. Nobody is an island, however much we might try to insulate ourselves. We are one human family. The implications of planetary connectedness are awesome. Energy follows thought. Energy follows feeling. The sense of separation only exists in our own minds and feeling natures that prefer to be absorbed in our own comfort. "Comfort", I remember reading many years ago, "is the graveyard of the Soul".

Many believe that the Christ will reappear in some form. I sometimes try to imagine what goes through His heart and mind as He faces and opens up to the human experience. If He is to return as many suggest, He cannot turn away. Perhaps His return can only occur through us. We are the mechanism of His facing up to the human situation. Or are we going to become His turning away? Will the Soul, the Christ within each of us, be allowed to find expression? The choice, I think, is *ours*.

Can we open our hearts to the collective human experience? Dare we open our hearts to the collective human experience? These are times that try our hearts and Souls to the limit, yes. That seems part of the deal as we move into the next millennium. Human hearts are awakening and it hurts. I always think of the rose bud, tearing itself apart so that it may unfold and reveal its hidden beauty for all to see. Many hearts remain tight, desperately trying not to burst under the pressure to open up. Yet as the rose bud must open in due season so must the human heart if we are to live to our potential as human beings. The closed heart enables the individual to remain insensitive to the plight and suffering of others. It remains closed to protect the individual from the hurt that will follow if they seek to reach out to another who is in pain.

We have to forget ourselves. We have to stand open to the flow of unconditional love that is the nature of the Soul and the energy of the heart. We have to find ways to cope with the hurt that it will bring us as we enter into truly heartfelt communion with our sisters and brothers everywhere. We have to love.

We surely live in the time of the call to love.

Part 4

Collaboration — the Workshops

by Richard and Lynn

When you stand in front of a mirror, what do you see?
You see a reflection of yourself.
In the same way, when we bring ourselves into the dance
we see ourselves reflected in it.
Yet it is more than a reflection:
it is a direct experience of who we are and how we function

Dancing the Sevenfold Energies of Life

Richard

The whole of life is a dance. The Seven Rays are a representation of the energies of life that affect us at every moment, at different periods of our lives and in different circumstances. Sacred Dance is a representation of these same energies borne out of the needs of communities around the world to express the aspects of life that are most dear to them or that affect them the most.

The dances are a means of living out important and powerful experiences in life. These same experiences are influenced by the Seven Rays. Our reaction to them depends on which Ray energies we choose to bring into play. Both are ways of understanding our life and experiencing it more fully, of gaining greater self-knowledge and awareness. Could we dovetail them together?

Combining worlds of experience

The idea began to take form that first evening we spent together. It germinated, and just under a year later came to fruition. By this time Lynn's scant knowledge of the Rays had expanded and I had become an 'addicted' circle dancer. We were entering each other's worlds and finding nourishment there; it was a great lesson for us both. We can so easily become fixed into a familiar world of interests and activities. We have been struck by how the overlapping of two very different areas can release tremendous creativity and fresh insight.

Many months prior to our first workshop, we started to compile a list of dances and the type of energy which they seemed to us to express. At the final planning session we discovered a pattern that until then had remained hidden. For each of the Rays at least one of the dances we had chosen involved movement into the centre of the circle. That movement was very different in each instance. We began to realise that the centre represented the focus of our aspiration, the goal of our endeavours however we might wish to define it; the way we approached it in dance became an expression of the spiritual journey of those influenced by that Ray energy. This was really exciting; we were touching on something quite unexpected.

Dancing the Rays

For example, one of the dances we use for the First Ray of Will or Power is Issos, a sun dance from Thrace. In this there is a very forceful stride into the centre; it is totally single-minded in its approach and nothing could divert it. The movement involves a definite push forward. It also has a powerful simplicity. These factors we felt made it very representative of some aspects of the energy of the first Ray. We use a quite different dance to experience its destructive face.

The Second Ray of Love-Wisdom, by comparison, has a quality of quiet persistence in its pursuit of its goal. We selected a gentle Yugoslavian dance which moves diagonally towards the centre. There is no pressure or push: what is experienced is a build up of momentum towards the goal, just the quiet yet firm persuasion of love/wisdom. It is as if the centre pulls us with a magnetic attraction.

For the Third Ray of Active Intelligence and Adaptability we dance Lamiita, a Romanian dance full of activity, which progresses towards the centre with a slightly complex weaving action. This is typical of the third Ray, which is an extremely active energy. It is also very much the Ray of the weaver, of versatility and adaptability. In this dance we put our energy into weaving our way towards our goal. Our second dance is also very active with a greater variety of steps, which requires us to keep moving in many different ways. It is a bit like whole-body juggling. We sometimes talk of this energy as being that of the tap-dancing executive — always on the move, always into this and that and everything else with mobile phones, faxes and every communication device you can imagine active at the same time. Yet with all the movement and juggling between one thing and the next, what is actually achieved? There is a third Ray type that cannot find the stillness needed to actually hold a focus long enough to create something tangible. It is always valuable in these dances to observe the centre of the circle, which never moves, but waits patiently and silently while we rush around it in all directions.

As you can imagine, the remaining four Rays (the Fourth Ray of Harmony through Conflict, of Beauty and Art; the Fifth Ray of Concrete Knowledge and Science; the Sixth Ray of Devotion and Idealism and the Seventh Ray of Ceremonial Order and Ritual) provide a further wealth of material with which to work. For the fourth Ray we concentrate on the quality of beauty as a way of spiritual growth and how we sometimes have to experience conflict in ourselves as part of the process of moving forward. We have chosen a beautiful, rhythmic dance set to the sound of a flute: it carries a powerful feeling of harmony, balance and artistic movement. The second dance we use is a favourite from Israel, Tsadik Katamar, sometimes referred to as The Wise Man and the Fool. The dance (although not the song) tells the tale of the different paths to enlightenment. The person who is wise just takes four steps and is there. The fool goes forwards, backwards, and round in a circle before finally getting there. Some say the fool has more fun on the journey! However, what it illustrates for people is how they handle confusion and conflict. It is a great dance to become entangled in: some people find they handle the difficulty by giving up, others use humour to cope, others refuse to be beaten and struggle on albeit with gritted teeth. Still others find it a challenge that they feel alive to. Isn't all this just like life? We all handle conflict in different ways — run away, fight back, hang in there doggedly, laugh it off but feel uncomfortable about it inside.

The fifth Ray suggests a mindful and methodical approach and has proved for us to be the most difficult energy to find dances for. However, we have one that requires you to stand upright and to move with a quality of mindfulness of your movements slowly around the circle. To complement this we have a dance that symbolises the scientific struggle in the pursuit of truth, going round looking for a place to start, methodical steps forward, a step back to review and reassess before further steps forward, final achievement and then start all over again with something else.

With the sixth Ray we seek to capture the dedication and devotion of the pilgrim in a dance that moves assuredly to a piece of 13th century Catalonian music. Pilgrims in this dance have their faces set towards their goal. It has almost a crusading feel to it which some are comfortable with, others not. To complement this we use a South American hymn, which touches the heart as the single voice hauntingly sings. The dance represents aspiration and reaching up before turning to give it out into the world. We also move in silent, individual reflection with our arms forming a cross over our hearts. The devotional attitude comes through strongly. We end at the centre of the circle, arms raised looking towards heaven in adoration, seeking inspiration.

The seventh Ray gives us an opportunity to experience the power of the ritualistic aspect of dance, and of life. We have changed this section on a number of occasions. We began with the Soweto Earth Dance, a powerful ritual yet somehow it did not feel exactly what we wanted. We have since begun to use a dance involving a strong rhythm, clapping, and hand movements that indicate the drawing down of energy. The latter is important as, whilst the sixth Ray influence encourages aspiration and reaching up, seventh Ray energy is about drawing down and giving out; if you like it is the bringing of spirit down into relationship with, and expression through, matter. It has a wonderful ordered feel to it.

Finally we offer a dance set to a Taizé chant that gives us space as individuals and allows us to join with the group in our ritualistic movement. The repetition of the chant and the movement combine to create an experience which for us reflects a quality of the seventh Ray. The aptly-named Dance of Unity provides us with a ceremonial end to our journey through the Seven Rays.

We must make it clear that we are not suggesting that our dances are in any way 'official' Seven Ray dances. They are the ones that we find help people to explore these energies. The Rays have many faces and would need many dances to capture them all. What is exciting, though, is that dance enables us to communicate with our own nature and with other people without the use of words.

The workshop experience

The first workshop brought together people who were entirely new to Sacred Dance, those who had no knowledge of the Seven Rays and even some for whom both were new. All were seeking to come to a fuller understanding of themselves and their life. We called it 'Energies of Life — Dance and the Seven Rays'. The whole of life is a dance, dance expresses life, the Rays are the energy of life.

The day went well and there was a lively discussion at the end about the dances we had suggested, the concept and qualities of the Seven Rays and how they interweave to produce the rich pattern of life. It seems important in our current world to introduce new ways of relating to the energies by which we are surrounded. Old patterns are changing and there is a need for people to experience for themselves rather than obtaining their knowledge only from books. Dance is a wonderful medium for this to take place. People remember how they felt while they were dancing, the type of energy that was active and the differing effects of the movements. The knowledge has been assimilated in the body, it has been experienced. The pattern of the dances has been internalised and at least part of the energy of each Ray is known at a level other than that of the mind.

Since that first workshop the title has evolved into 'Dancing the Sevenfold Energies of Life'.

The sevenfold circle

The circle is a powerful symbol. It contains, represents, and is, the whole. Being part of a circle can therefore have a potent effect. We enter the world of the symbol. It is fascinating how in the dance we can experience the simultaneity of being both an individual and part of a group. In the circle we are all equal. There is no separation although we have the space to experience our individuality. The journey into the centre becomes symbolic of the group nature of spiritual growth, yet we take responsibility within the group for our own movement.

The idea of combining dance and the Seven Rays continues to evolve. It is by no means final. If it provides a medium through which people can grow and there is a demand for this kind of approach, then it is sure to develop further. We have run this workshop over one and two days, in three-hour sessions across a number of days and in a whole variety of settings. What is so fascinating is how each experience is different. The circle is always made up of a different combination of people, each bringing their own energies to bear upon the experience.

Sometimes one particular Ray energy will come to the fore and the group will want to re-experience the dance and the feelings that it brings up. On other occasions certain Ray energies are just anathema to the group. Nobody wants to know them. Our attention was drawn to this with one group when dancing the energy of the first Ray. They simply did not like it, the thought of a destructive and powerful energy was not what they wanted to be near. Yet for us there has to be destruction (a face of the first Ray), and its complement, building and creation (a quality of the second Ray). Wholeness is literally this. We cannot afford to limit ourselves to what we feel comfortable with. Surely we need to explore, and be prepared to participate in, all aspects of creation, learning to do so under the wise prompting of the Soul nature.

There was the woman who in a first Ray dance, which involves a strong placing of the foot on the ground was really struggling. "I just could not put my foot down", she said. You could almost see the light bulb coming on over her head: "That's me isn't it? It's my life pattern," she admitted, as she saw herself reflected in this one movement. It had taken the experience of the dance to enable her to gain this insight, thereby offering her the opportunity to question the habit of a lifetime.

Another participant realised how important the active energy associated with the third Ray was for her. "I've been seeking peace all along. But I really enjoyed that dance; I feel alive and vitalised. I think now that I need more of that in my life." She could not fill her life with it, that would be too much, but at present there was none and she needed to explore how to integrate it into her weekly routine. Who knows, maybe by doing this she will open up other possibilities as she works more with this energy.

What of our own experiences? We have found that, however often we run this workshop, we still gain fresh insights into ourselves each time. Recently, Lynn had a very powerful realisation about a relationship with which she was struggling. As she revealed in the group discussion, "During the first and second Ray dances I suddenly knew where the problem lay: I was focusing on a negative aspect of the second Ray — the poor me, I am of no value. I need to apply a little of the first Ray confidence and direction." Since then this relationship has changed for her: she tells me, "I now feel able to express my real self with confidence. I now feel respected and heard." Is it surprising that the other person involved seems to have changed as well?

Whilst we normally run this workshop over one or two days, we have extended it across a week providing more space for people to look at themselves in the light of the Seven Rays. We often need time (and space) to absorb, reflect on and make sense of our experiences, something we can lose sight of in the hectic culture of 'busyness' and 'quick-fix' that seems to pervade western society.

Visualisation

In all our work we employ the use of visualisation to complement and reinforce the experience gained in the dance. One that we use in this workshop places a specific focus on the colour and the qualities of the second Ray of Love-Wisdom. It aims to enable the individual to approach this energy, initially at least, in a way that does not involve the interpretation of words. Imagining colour enables us to establish a vibration on subtle levels without it becoming cluttered up with mental concepts. Once the colour is being held clearly *then* the words are used to provide the mental focus.

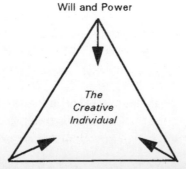

Figure 8.
The triangle of creativity

In another visualisation we emphasise the interaction of the first, second and third Rays within the creative process. These three energies might be regarded as forming a triangle with the individual at the centre drawing on the different energies at different stages of the creative process (Figure 8).

Beginning with the initiating impulse of the first Ray to enable clarity and direction as the initial idea is formulated, through the building and magnetic note of the second Ray in which the blueprint of the eventual form is constructed, we add the creative and intelligent force of the third Ray to generate the final form. What is produced has thus been moulded to the blueprint and is an expression of the original creative impulse and intent. This way of working with creativity is basic and can be applied to any situation. In the workshop a short visualisation takes us through these three stages, allowing participants the opportunity to apply them to a project or an idea in which they themselves have an interest.

Seven Rays visualisation

The final visualisation concerns the image that links us to the title of this book — the sevenfold circle. It involves the creative imagining of a seven-spoked wheel, each spoke carrying a particular stream of Ray energy with ourselves at the centre (see Figure 9).

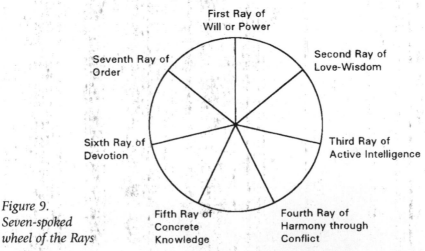

*Figure 9.
Seven-spoked
wheel of the Rays*

Sit in a relaxed position and let your breathing become steady and rhythmic. Be aware of yourself, of your boundaries and of the strength of your own still centre deep within. Imagine that you are sitting at the centre of a seven-spoked wheel. You are the hub. Each spoke conveys a stream of energy:

Spoke 1 — energy of will or power.
Allow yourself to experience where and how the energy touches you. Affirm to yourself the presence of the power and will that you intend to express.

Spoke 2 — energy of love-wisdom.
Allow yourself to experience where and how the energy touches you. Sense yourself attracting the quality of love and wisdom that you aspire to express.

Spoke 3 — energy of active intelligence and adaptability.
Allow yourself to experience where and how the energy touches you. Imagine this energy being woven into the very fabric of your nature.

Spoke 4 — energy of harmony through conflict, of beauty and art.
Allow yourself to experience where and how the energy touches you. Sense the emergence of harmony and beauty through your own art of living.

Spoke 5 — energy of concrete knowledge and science.
Allow yourself to experience where and how the energy touches you. Reflect on the quality of knowledge and scientific thought that you seek to grasp with your own mind.

Spoke 6 — energy of devotion and idealism.
Allow yourself to experience where and how the energy touches you. Feel the presence of devotion and idealism within yourself and consider its nature and direction.

Spoke 7 — energy of ritual and order.
Allow yourself to experience where and how the energy touches you. Visualise a new order within your life that is more deeply expressive of the Soul nature.

Seven streams of energy, some we feel more closely akin to than others. Yet we must learn, through the cycles of time, to master them all and dedicate their use in service of the Greater Good.

Still within the seven-spoked wheel, and holding a state of spiritual poise, sense the wheel beginning to spin; as it does so, the energy streams out from the seven points at the circumference, like a catherine wheel, spinning out into the world. Thus we stand.

Let the spinning slow to a stop. Draw in to your physical body and make a point of noting the solid ground beneath you and the sounds around you. Think of the room and the people who are with you in the group. Be aware of your breathing and, in your own time, open your eyes and smile across the circle. You may wish to have a stretch and to feel the presence of your physical self.

Each visualisation should be brief, no more than 15 minutes. It is used to help to anchor the experience of the day within the person and is very thoughtful. Through its use we are seeking clarification and affirmation. It rounds off the day, affording us all the opportunity to affirm what the different energies mean to us, in terms of our own experiences and spheres of work, responsibility and service.

It is also important to point out that the value of this workshop, as with all the others, is in the relationship that is established during the course of the time that we are together. The group bond that is created is a crucial factor. It is this experience that has encouraged us to apply our way of working to teambuilding (described in the appendices). In our *Self Awareness in Dance* workshops we find that learning and insight come through the intra- and inter-personal relationships within the group relationship. As we compare and contrast our own process of engagement within the group we gain fresh insight into how and who we are. In seeking clarity on this we prepare ourselves to face more effectively the challenges, the demands and the opportunities that life presents to us.

Dancing the Zodiac: the Soul's Journey to Greater Light

Richard

It is strange how connections run from the past to bring immense significance in the present and future. It was back in the 1980s that I attended a gathering of people from East and West Europe in Brighton. At the time I was working for the Lucis Trust, for whom I was running a stand. One of the people I met was Margot Graham from Poland who was over to discuss some translation work for the Lucis Trust, in particular the *Triangles Bulletin*.[16] We got on really well and shared some time during her stay. Funnily enough it was in Brighton at that gathering that I had my first contact with Sacred Circle Dance too!

A few years later, when Lynn and I had devised our first workshop, I wrote to Margot to tell her about the recent changes in my life. We were very soon invited to participate in a summer camp in Poland. At the time we only had our Seven Rays workshop to offer. Margot is an astrologer, so naturally enough we thought that this might be a good theme to explore in dance.

We chose to approach it from the angle of esoteric astrology, which is quite different in many respects from a purely horoscope approach. The idea is that we come under different signs of the zodiac as we move along our evolutionary path. What we wanted to get across was that we work with energies associated with these different signs at particular stages on the path of development. To begin with, the influence of the signs drives consciousness towards involvement in matter. Then, as we move away from a material emphasis, the energies drive our consciousness towards expansion and liberation from matter.

We felt we could not cover all of this in one workshop, that we would have to somehow combine the drive downwards into form and material identity, with the struggle to find our true selves and eventual liberation. What we created is, to the purist, a distortion, yet at the same time it is, we believe, a valuable introduction to an astrological perspective that can be extremely difficult to grasp — the idea that the energies of the zodiacal signs govern different stages on the path of evolution. This is *esoteric* or *Soul-centred astrology*.

In the workshop we begin with a dance that expresses the endless chain of rebirth. We move round the circle in a methodical and almost automatic manner as if driven along by an unseen force, pausing to step into the centre of the circle (symbolically taking form) and then stepping back out to the turning wheel. And so it continues, in, out and move along. Like life. Or at least, this is how it can seem until we realise ourselves to be conscious and creative participants in the process; then the experience is radically altered. After this introductory dance we move into our journey around the zodiacal wheel (Figure 10).

---

16.   Triangles is a meditation network in which people agree to link with each other in thought each day in threes, to visualise and create triangles of light and goodwill as an act of world service.

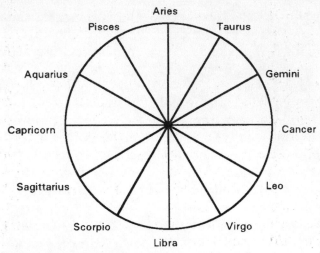

Figure 10. The zodiacal wheel

We take a journey that involves a descent of consciousness into form, the development of that consciousness within the form and then a final stage

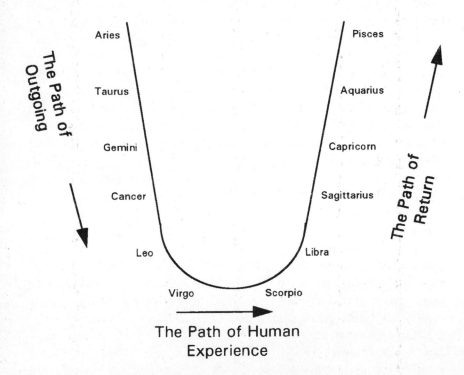

Figure 11. The zodiacal journey

that is concerned with liberation from form (Figure 11).

Aries

We begin with Aries, sign of commencement and new beginnings. Aries governs thought and the initiation of ideas. All of creation proceeds out of thought, whether we are considering Divine thought behind the greater creative processes of the cosmos, or the creativity of the individual human being. Some people are full of ideas, but never seem to be able to find the creative expression that enables them to take form. Others seem to put ideas into practice as if it was as natural as breathing. In fact, in reality, it *is* as natural as breathing! Yet, in our modern, technological world where so many decisions are taken for us, it is actually easy to lose touch with our innate ability to initiate and act on our own ideas. The same can happen to those living under centralised and totalitarian political systems. The ability is lost and it is a real struggle to re-introduce it.

In terms of our zodiacal journey we might think of the Aries experience as being linked to the decision to incarnate. This approach to astrology assumes and accepts the reality of rebirth. Under the influence of Aries the decision is taken to proceed once more into form. The greater Self (the Soul) induces the lesser self (the spark of human consciousness) to seek to clothe itself in matter. The descent begins.

We use a dance to symbolise this steady movement down into matter, into the darkness. We move to the left, which symbolises this process and we trace the shape of the cross with our feet. We are symbolically and in reality creating a cross in matter. This cross we might consider to be the four-fold human personality comprising physical, etheric, emotional and mental aspects. In Aries we engage with the plane of the mind. The Soul sounds its note with the words: *I come forth and from the plane of mind, I rule.*

Taurus

The next sign is Taurus, symbolised by the bull, and very much concerned with desire and emotion. The spark of consciousness descends further into the plane of emotional living, of feeling and reaction. It is a place of great glamour where our experiences can be dominated and distorted by separative feeling-based reactions. 'Glamour' denotes a distortion generated by the strong feeling currents that swirl through the astral plane; we can find ourselves resonating to their seductive note and being swept along by them.

The doorway to the emotional plane is the solar plexus centre. We know what it is like when our feelings are churned up; we feel them in our stomach. When this centre is open and active, but not controlled, we can so easily be swept by powerful feelings which, as they pour into us, feel as if they are truly our own. We get caught up in them. We find it difficult to stand back and to gain a sense of proportion about what is happening.

The astral plane is also the plane of desire: so much of the human experience in our world today is rooted in selfish and separative desire. It is easy to tune into this and to lose touch with clear thinking. In the workshop we use a dance that takes us on a journey into (and out of) the labyrinth. Labyrinths and mazes provide us with symbolic journeys into the underworld, into the dark, in order that we might return into the light enriched from the fruit of that experience.

Our desire carries us into the labyrinth, into the life of material living. We lose sight of our true inner direction. We become caught up in the maze of illusion and glamour that we create through the endless pursuit of happiness, unaware that in life all intent that is rooted in desire will of necessity give us both that which we seek, and its built-in opposite. Desirelessness is a great and commanding ideal. We would each do well to consider our lives from the angle of this great quality.

As with all the signs, the associated energies, as well as driving us into form, provide us with the means of release. The built-in opposite once again. The call of the Soul in Taurus is: *I see and when the Eye is opened, all is light.* The eye of the bull is at first pointed only towards its desire. In time, and through learning, desire will be transmuted into aspiration towards the finer things of the spirit. When the eye opens to this goal, greater light pours forth and truth is seen, but the veils of glamour must be pierced, and the eye on opening must be of singular intent.

In our journey we have clothed ourselves in mental and emotional matter. We have already touched on duality, and this aspect of creation asserts itself as we journey under the influence of Gemini, symbolised by the twins.

Gemini

Gemini brings us choice, the 'this or that' sign; we seem to find ourselves pulled first one way, then the other. It brings great fluidity and the tendency to flit from one experience to another. We symbolise this in the dance for this sign with occasional moments of steadiness before moving off again wherever our fancy takes us. It is so difficult to stay focused.

We are full of energy and susceptibility to the power of the desire nature.

In Gemini we take on the energy body, the etheric, the subtle energy matrix that underlies the physical form. The ancients knew this well; for instance, in the healing arts through such traditions as acupuncture. The physical body is driven by the energy currents within the etheric body. These are largely governed by our thought and emotional life. When our thoughts and feelings are 'knotted up', distortions occur in the etheric energy flow and we are more likely to succumb to disease.

From a deeper perspective, Gemini is also about the relationship between the Soul and its form, between the spiritual self and the human personality through which it seeks expression. Eventual achievement in Gemini is concerned with bringing the separative personality under the Soul's direction and influence. In this sign the Soul calls forth: *I recognise my other self and in the waning of that self I grow and glow.* The other self is the separative human personality as a state of consciousness. The one thing more than anything else that we need to rid ourselves of in this world is the sense of separateness. It is not real. It distorts the flow of force and energy through the human family across the planet. Hence the social diseases of poverty, homelessness and starvation. Energy does not flow equably where separative identity dominates. The diseases of the body are so often reflections of the same law.

We hear talk of a global community. Are we a global community? Have we grasped the basic essentials of what this really means, 'global common-unity'? Is this what we see in our world? Do we not see separateness and selfishness ravishing the human spirit, and the desire for material well-being, for comfort, distorting the natural economic flow which should follow the guiding principle of sharing? I do not think we can have global community until our minds and our hearts grasp what it actually means. Then we can explore how to live it. There are many experiments and many who are seeking to make this a reality. I believe that all who are working for right human relations, for freedom and responsibility and who shun exploitation and self-interest whatever glossy form it is dressed in, need and deserve our support and encouragement.

Cancer

So we move on to Cancer, the sign of mass experience and mass consciousness. Under the influence of this energy the individual spark of consciousness takes form and enters into the human experience. However, at this stage on the journey the individual is very much conditioned by mass movement, by the prevailing thought and feeling currents that are around him or her. Cancer as it governs this stage is not concerned with self-consciousness. It is much more the mass experience and we use a dance that requires us to move fast and in such close contact with the people on either side of us that we have little room or scope for individual expression. The circle moves and we have to move with it. We are unable to make any other choice for we are unaware that we *can* make any other choice.

Cancer is also the sign of the crab, of the person who carries their home around with them. This can mean that someone likes their own space, their own home, and home-making becomes their natural expression. It can of course run to extremes and become stifling and limiting. At the other end of the scale is the person who has awakened to self-consciousness and who now carries his or her own space through life. This may be thought of as a bubble that extends to our own boundaries of self. Some people have a very small and tight bubble, almost pressing against their skin. For other people it extends further. It is an interesting and valuable exercise to consider how far your bubble of space extends. How much of your home or your work environment does your bubble comfortably embrace, or is it squeezed by others and how does that affect you?

The keynote of the Soul in Cancer is *I build a lighted house and therein dwell*. This refers to a later stage of Cancerian influence as the individual builds his or her etheric energy field to carry Soul impulse. The Soul-infused etheric body is the lighted house. We seek to build this as individuals, we seek to build it collectively. As we each live more fully in a manner that reflects or expresses Soul impulse, the etheric energy matrix will be transformed and the sustaining energy patterns that underlie physical form will undergo refinement.

Visualisation (1) — The Path of Outgoing

The Journey into form
We affirm our essence as immortal Souls. As Sacred Flames of Light and Love, we observe the unceasing perpetual wheel of rebirth, preparing to enter once more into incarnation.

Aries
The idea of our new incarnation emerges and we put down a spark of consciousness, a spark of ourselves, into the world of thought. We journey down, as that spark into the dark, into matter, into form-life. We danced to the left carrying our cross

on our journey of descent. Aries is the sign in which the creative cycle is initiated, involution begins. It is the sign of creative thought — all creation originates from the realm of ideas.

Taurus

From mind to emotion, our spark of consciousness now enters the astral realm of feeling and desire. It is a labyrinth of illusion and glamour. We clothe ourselves in the substance of this fluid realm. We know that eventually desire must be transmuted into aspiration, but on the involutionary arc our desire is towards experience in form, towards the world of human feeling. Only on our return journey may we find a way through the labyrinth to release the 'bull of desire' that it might direct our aspiration towards greater light.

Gemini

We clothe ourselves in physical form and awaken to duality. We experience imbalance and the fluid tendency to flit from one experience to another, often seemingly opposites. One moment we have a certain stability, and the next we are off on another flight of fancy. We experience the duality of life as we move further into form under this zodiacal influence.

Cancer

Finally, through the door of Cancer, we enter into the world, into the form-life of humanity, into incarnation. Here we experience mass movement. The circle moves and we must go with it, no room for any sense of individuality as we are carried by the herd. Within the closed group there is also protection, a hard shell to conceal our own vulnerability. With little true self-consciousness we move from side to side, but do we ever seem to get anywhere? We experience a closeness, a certain security as the tide of mass expression pushes us along.

Leo

On our journey through the zodiac we next experience Leo, the sign which, *par excellence*, governs the emergence of the individual, self-conscious unit. This is the sign whose energy encourages the integration of the human personality — physical/etheric, emotional and mental natures — creating a powerful mechanism that may (or may not) be used to express Soul purpose.

Leo is about power — personal power — where it governs the emergence of the self-conscious unit from the mass consciousness of humanity. There is a difference between mass and group consciousness; the eventual goal for the self-conscious individual is to achieve group consciousness. We return to this in Aquarius. Mass consciousness operates at an instinctive level: group consciousness operates at the intuitive level. The two are often confused, but in reality they are, quite literally, poles apart.

Many people act out of a belief that the universe will somehow always direct them and they become like leaves in the wind with little or no personal intention or will in their lives. Whilst this can indeed carry them to where they need to be, they are not actually learning to be *conscious* participators in life. This is crucial because, in the final analysis, we are struggling to learn to become co-creators within the great scheme of things. We have to make choices and decisions and live through the experiences that follow from them. We have to learn to discriminate the real from the unreal; we do this largely through experimentation. Humanity has surely to move beyond instinctive living and begin to embrace Soul-centred living, to cultivate the infallible intuitive sense. Let us be clear, intuition is not hunching, it is not supported by frantic self-justification, or blaming others when things do not work out as we had envisioned! Intuition is a knowing that is rooted in Soul awareness and which is undistorted by personal reaction. In essence it is a faculty of the Soul, the power to perceive the truth of things without reasoning or analysis.

The power of the integrated personality imposes itself on life and experience. We use a dance that enables each participant to experience power in themselves, power over their own space and movement, power that is reflected in a certain majestic bearing. At the extreme end, Leo influence at this stage can lead to the emergence of the dictator. It will certainly produce forceful individuals and there are many in the world at this time. Yet we must look beyond the force and the power and grasp where it is flowing from (is their consciousness centred in the Soul or the separative self?) and where it is going to (the great test of motive that all must face in their endeavours).

The keynote of the Soul in Leo can seem curious: *I am That and That am I*. There are many interpretations but perhaps the simplest is that it is the Soul affirming that there is no longer separation between itself and the personality. The individual offers the personality nature as a vehicle of service to the Soul, and the Soul takes hold of it knowing that it can be relied on to respond with love and intelligence. This, however, comes later, for in our journey around the zodiac in dance we are emphasising the experience of the power of the integrated personality.

Virgo

With all the signs, we learn not only through engaging with their inherent qualities and influence, but also through the contrast in experience as we move from sign to sign. On our interpretation of the zodiacal wheel we regard Virgo as ruling the birth of the Christ-consciousness within the heart. What does this mean in words we can grasp?

We have just experienced the personal power of Leo, now we are called on to reorient our focus to another source of power, a much more potent source and certainly one that will outlast the transient personality. We are looking towards that first glimpse of the Soul nature, the Christ aspect that is present in each of us. Our use of the word 'Christ' is not strictly Christian, but refers to that immortal aspect of creation that is not only at the core of our being, but in a deeper sense *is* the core of our being. In Virgo we glimpse a higher, deeper, more loving and expansive possibility.

We symbolise this using a dance that takes us on an individual spiral journey. We look back into the past and we turn to face the future, giving ourselves the chance to feel the release of energy that this inevitably brings. So many of us are tied to the past, unable to free ourselves from old patterns of thought, reaction and behaviour. We will look at this more closely when we consider transition in another chapter. Dare we look to the future, to actually begin to think ahead towards the possibilities that we might bring into being?

Having made this turn symbolically in the dance we spiral down as if to reach down into ourselves, a form of grounding in our strictly human nature, only to then turn, reversing the spiral as we reach up into the light, towards our higher potential. We can only do this because we have cultivated sensitivity to the Soul nature, because we have begun to reject the material and selfish values that pervade our world and have recognised the need for something more, something more sustainable as a way of being.

The Soul's keynote in Virgo links heaven and earth and contains great potency as an affirmation: *I am the Mother and the Child. I, God, I, matter am.* The language may seem strange yet it contains a simple truth — that I, the Soul, the essence of my being, pervades all creation. That I include both the Mother aspect of creation and the Son. That I form a bridge between God and matter. I am the impulse that carries spirit into matter and through their relationship brings forth the Son — consciousness, the Christ principle. Under the influence of Virgo the flickering light of the Soul is sensed within the human heart, a new reality is touched and we are now confronted with a choice: the path of continued separation, or the path towards unity, connectedness and service.

Libra

Libra is the sign of balance, the energy that qualifies the experience of weighing up situations and choices. In our journey in dance we depict this sign in terms of the decision to be made between treading the spiritual path, or the material path. We have experienced the power of the personality in Leo, we have glimpsed and reached up towards the Christ light in Virgo, now we must choose the way ahead. The keynote of the Soul in this sign sums it up: *I choose the way which leads between the two great lines of force.*

What are these great lines? The pull of the opposites, the emotional forces that through our desire we engage with and which lock us into the treadmill of pleasure and pain.

The challenge lies in re-orienting desire into aspiration towards the spiritual nature, towards living a life of selfless service. Yet we are caught in a moment (that can last a lifetime) of transition and choice. Libra rules the interludes between activities. Therefore it rules our present time as we move towards and through the start of the next millennium, as we bridge between the Piscean and Aquarian ages. We live in an era of transition and, with the speed and intensity of life increasing, the pressure to adapt and change seemingly continuously is extremely pervasive.

We use a dance that requires us to feel the instability of balance, and its centredness when we actually find it and hold it with poise and equilibrium. The movement involves rising up on one leg on to our toes. For me, the classic Libran balance, the overhead balance with the fulcrum above, provides us with a symbol that we can gain much from exploring. The dishes on either side contain opposites, providing forces that act in opposition on the balance. The fulcrum above can be seen as the apex of a triangle, that unites and yet is more than the two lower points. This image we use in another of our workshops: 'Beyond Balance — Towards Complementarity'.

Another way of viewing the Libran balance is to consider one dish as containing the sum total of the separative nature, the other the sum total of Soul-centred expression. Our lives are literally held in the balance, as is our choice for future emphasis.

So Libra provides us with a choice on our journey. Are we ready to face the challenge of living the spiritual life? Have our hearts opened to the Soul allowing us to seek a way that will take us clear of separative and materialistic living? Or is the desire life still dominant, binding us through its attractive force to further material experience? In Libra we truly enter the balance on our journey and we make our choice.

When our choice is to travel the spiritual path we enter on a new phase of our journey. Now our attention is towards the light, towards the Soul and reunion with our immortal selves. But are we really committed? Do we have the wherewithal to make this journey? There is an obstruction on the path and it is a familiar face — our own. It is an ageless truism that on each bend of the spiritual path we meet ourselves, the separative tendencies that are lodged within our physical, emotional and mental natures, the appetites of the lower self.

Scorpio

Thus we enter under the influence of Scorpio, the sign of trial and testing. On our journey in dance we are called on to confront the separative self. In the Hercules myth that Alice Bailey links to this sign,[17] Hercules is called upon to slay a nine-headed hydra. Each head represents an appetite of the separative personality:

Physical life
1. Sex 2. Comfort 3. Money

Emotional life
4. Fear 5. Hatred 6. Desire for power

Thought life
7. Pride 8. Separativeness 9. Cruelty

He finds that as he cuts off one head, two grow in its place. He cannot root out the separateness one part at a time. His only practical approach is to confront it whole. He kneels (symbolising his humility) and lifts the hydra out of the mud, breaking its attachment to earth, raising it into the light where it dies from lack of nourishment. As the others droop, Hercules sees the mystical head which he then severs.

For us, this need to rise by kneeling is important. We cannot fight force with force on its own level, but rather must carry it into another realm. The hydra could not sustain itself when raised into the light, the separative tendencies of the personal self become unsustainable in the inclusive light of the Soul. This basic idea is crucial for our world at this time. Separateness is rampant. Yet it is only sustained because we feed it through our own separative attitudes and actions.

As we learn to live free of separation we will find separateness as a prevailing attitude will wither. It is inherently unsustainable where co-operation and community is being fostered. Yes, there will be a raging

17 . Alice A Bailey, *The Labours of Hercules* (Lucis Press Ltd, London) pp. 69–71.

battle, we see it now in our world. We see separative attitudes behind exploitation and the refusal to resolve poverty, disease and homelessness. We, humanity, under the influence of Libra, are being called to choose our way ahead in the midst of the battle. Under Scorpio we must face the challenge of rooting out separateness, having made our choice.

The keynote of the Soul in Scorpio runs: *Warrior am I, and from the battle I emerge triumphant.* Yes, we are called upon to be warriors. Does this seem strange when there is so much talk of peace? Peace is not the solution to our problems. You cannot create peace, you can only create conditions in which peace can flourish. Hence the emphasis on the concept of the 'Peace Process'. Peace emerges finally, but not initially. We want it because we do not want war. This is not the answer.

What will bring peace is wanting to live in right relationship with people and the planet. What will bring peace is the destruction of the separative attitudes that have for too long governed human interaction. What will bring peace is a willingness to forget ourselves in service of the common good thus forging an atmosphere of goodwill. Then and only then, does peace have a chance. Then and only then, can peace become a sustainable fact on Earth.

* * *

Visualisation (2) — The Path of Human Experience

The Experience and Mastery of our Sense of Personal Identity

Leo
We affirm our potency as powerful and integrated personalities. We experience the individual forcefulness of Leo. Here there is an opportunity to acknowledge a sense of our own personal power. Still in the group, but now with time and space for ourselves. Yet, can we begin to sense how limiting this separative individuality can be as we roar through life, imposing our needs on others and the environment around us?

Virgo
We have nurtured our form nature, yet it is unsatisfying. In Virgo comes an opportunity to sense that deeper reality, that touch of the Christ impulse which we must now nurture and protect. The past has brought us to the present. We are caught between the past and the future. The past, should we cling to it, we experience as a block to our progress. Can we turn away from it and, by so doing, affirm our reality in the present, and free ourselves

to spiral up towards the Christ nature æ the Soul? Can we, as the separative spark, dimly sense the presence of that Sacred Flame deep within that we left behind on the descent in Aries?

Libra

Time to reflect and weigh-up the journey so far. An interlude in which to balance our experiences and to make our choices. As we raise ourselves up on tip-toe we may rock to and fro, experiencing the vulnerability of our instability and the need for balance. Our future is now truly in the balance. Will we swing towards a cycle of spiritual striving, accepting the tests and trials that will surely follow this decision, or choose to return, once more, into the round of material experience, driven by unfulfilled desires? Will the light of the Soul inspire a wise choice?

Scorpio

And so into battle as the warrior, yet it is not ourselves as personalities that undertake the struggle, but the Soul nature to which we are developing increasing sensitivity. Can we, as Souls, conquer our personal natures, symbolised by the many-headed hydra of selfish and separative living? We think of the separative tendencies within us and imagine ourselves raising them into the light. We rise by kneeling, we grow through humility. We kneel and thus lift the hydra, unearthing it and allowing a Greater Light to weaken it to death. We take our stand as spiritual warriors.

Sagittarius

We enter the final phase of the journey around the zodiac, the four signs that take us through the experience of initiation, towards the responsibility of world service and eventual liberation from earthly experience. Initiation is often spoken of in hushed tones. Yet it need not be so. It is simply a ceremony that marks the individual (or group) readiness to shoulder greater responsibility in service to the Divine Plan. Those who are truly initiate do not make fantastic claims or promote their level of initiation as a basis on which to judge the wisdom of their teachings. Concerns as to who is, or who is not, initiate, is a waste of precious time that could be much better used in serving the immediate need of humanity.

We can find the energy of Sagittarius expressing itself in many areas of life, but what distinguishes it from the idealistic urge that is often coloured by emotion and desire is that there is a clear mental grasp of the nature and purpose of the journey being taken. Thought is present.

Sagittarius is a fire sign, a sign of direction and purpose. In our workshop we use a fire dance that is extremely lively and purposeful. The energy is that of goal-oriented living. The tests and trials have been met in Scorpio and now the urge is to drive on towards Greater Light.

Desire for personal goals and achievements are transmuted into a fiery aspiration towards the spirit. There is no sense of going back now, indeed the path behind is probably no longer available. Forward, ever forward, driven by knowing what must be undertaken and achieved.

The keynote of the Soul in Sagittarius expresses the direction and purposefulness of the sign: *I see the goal. I reach that goal, and then I see another.* Such is the way of evolution. We move from goal to goal and in our attainment lies the opportunity to glimpse a further horizon, another goal to be worked for and achieved. In terms of spiritual growth we might relate this to a path that takes us towards greater truth. Each time we see a little more and our minds awaken more fully to the light of the intuition, we engage with truth and we are called on to live what we now know. Knowledge brings responsibility. Then, having demonstrated our ability to apprehend truth and apply it wisely, we see that farther horizon. So we move on, step by step, into the light, into greater awareness of reality. Initiation, in the final analysis, is entry into the light of truth. Each successive initiation marks an expansion of consciousness and indicates a readiness to shoulder greater responsibility in service.

Capricorn

The sign of the crocodile, the goat and the unicorn, depending on whether your life is centred in wallowing in the mud and water of emotional living, concerned with climbing steep, rocky challenges with dogged determination or whether your one-pointedness has brought you to the final achievement of standing on the apex of the mountain of initiation. On our journey around the zodiac we represent the goat using a wonderful Israeli dance that is all about climbing the Golan Heights. If you have not been to Israel, this mountain range runs along and beyond the Sea of Galilee creating a wonderful backdrop. In the dance we zig-zag up the mountain, pausing at times to catch our breath, or maybe to reflect on our achievement and the nature of the next step before us. Eventually we reach the summit, the goat becomes the wondrous unicorn, the single horn representing singleness of purpose that has become integrated into the individual who has achieved — no longer personal determination but now a purposeful will.

The Soul in Capricorn sounds its keynote with the words: *Lost am I in light supernal, yet on that light I turn my back*. We lose our personal identity within this greater light that is of the Soul. A fusion takes place and whilst we do not lose our individuality, we begin to realise the meaning of unity. Yet we cannot remain on the summit. Many consider the climbing of the mountain marks final achievement but this is not so. We reach the heights, we experience the ecstasy of spiritual union, but if this was the end then somehow it would make a mockery of creation. No, initiation is not a way of escape. It is a path that brings us the opportunity to love and serve more wisely, more intelligently, and more practically in line with divine intention.

At the summit in Capricorn we are called to turn and travel back into the valley, back down towards struggling humanity to aid others on their journey towards the light, or perhaps to point the way to those who have not even begun to travel this path in a conscious sense. It reminds me of the images people describe in the near-death experience. I do not suggest that such experiences are an indication of initiation, but there is often an impression of entering a region of light, followed by a sense of losing something precious as the individual identity is drawn back into form, clothed again in substance to become embroiled once more in the drama of human living. For some people it is a choice that they themselves make, for others it is as though a force pulls them back inexorably into the world of matter.

So the individual goes down the mountain, turning their back on the light, not to ignore it, but in a sense to carry it with them. They become as light-bearers. I think this also needs some clarification. We hear so much of light-workers and light-bearers in certain quarters and it always seems to be spoken in hushed tones. The true light-bearer makes no claim as to status. He or she serves. Service rendered *is* their reward. Personal acclamation is not important. As we struggle to free ourselves from the dominance of emotional living we must also free ourselves from the urge to sit in awe at the feet of others and to bask in our favoured close proximity. There is only one master that matters, the Soul within. Until we have found that there is little use in seeking elsewhere. And when we have found it, we will have no urge to seek elsewhere.

One of the planets associated with Capricorn is Saturn which many see as an enemy somehow, for to them it symbolises karmic retribution. Yet on a higher turn of the spiral Saturn is perceived as a friendly influence, stimulating the experiences that we need that will enable us to climb the mountain. This might be seen as a mountain of karma for us to surmount — so-called good and bad (though in truth it has neither label outside the emotionally driven human mind) — enabling us in time to be free of personal indebtedness to the great law of cause and effect. In Capricorn we reach the point where we free ourselves from Saturn's karmic touch.

Aquarius

The return journey to the valley of human experience requires us to carry light into the world. Selfless service is the essence of Aquarius, of reaching up or within in order to give out. The sense of separateness has faded and the individual spark of consciousness, that began its descent back in Aries, now knows what it is to be united with the Soul, the flame, the group-consciousness that had been obscured through cycles of separative and individual living.

We are currently in transition from an era ruled by Pisces towards one governed by Aquarius. When will it happen? Who knows? Who cares? It really does not matter and if people want to argue about dates and produce prophecies that can never be proved, then so be it. What seems to be important is to place emphasis on the special qualities associated with this sign, and the foremost of these is *service*.

Service is the natural expression of the spiritual Self, the true Self, the Soul. The keynote of the Soul in Aquarius is: *Water of Life am I, poured forth for thirsty men*. In our journey in dance through the signs of the zodiac we represent the Aquarian impulse of service and carrying the waters of Life out into the world. We symbolically bring water from the centre of the circle, turn, and face outwards. For this is the higher expression of Aquarius. It governs our journey back down from the mountain, from that high point reached in Capricorn, in which we symbolically and in truth carry with us the waters of Life to be given through service to humanity. No longer are our energies devoted to serving the cause of the separative desire-life. Now our energies are directed in service, in creating a life that will bring hope and direction to others.

Aquarius is also linked to the development of group consciousness. It is interesting to note that this is the opposite sign to Leo, sign of individuality and self-consciousness. We can gain much by considering the opposite signs as complements or contrasts within a single process. In a real sense we cannot become group conscious without passing through a stage of self-consciousness. We have to realise our personal identity and to then carry this on our journey towards Greater Light. As we enter into communion with the Soul our sense of self-consciousness undergoes transformation. The sense of separateness is faced and rooted out, enabling us to realise a sense of connectedness and group purpose.

What do we mean by 'group consciousness'? We are talking essentially about Soul-consciousness, or identification with the Real Self which does not contain the separative sense that in human form we are conditioned and accustomed to accepting as reality. It also means that we can work in line with a greater purpose, for our own personal interests and enthusiasms take second place to the demands of the group intent. Our personal and often petty self-will is no longer the driving force behind our lives. We realise the importance of motive and under Soul impression our motive is ever rooted in harmlessness, self-forgetfulness and a joyful willingness to love and serve.

We see in our world so many groups dedicated to service, from the large-scale international organisations working to raise the human condition and the state of the planet, right through to the local community-based organisations. Many feel depressed by the scale of need on our planet. The reality is that there are today more men and women of goodwill engaged in service, in working for the welfare of human beings, other forms of life on our planet and the Earth itself than ever before in human history. This is an expression of the awakening human heart and we must be encouraged by it and seek inspiration to participate ourselves in the planetary network of service.

Pisces

The final sign in our journey is one of liberation and of flying free from the endless cycle of rebirth. It is the sign of the world saviour, of the individual who has become a living thread of consciousness between heaven and earth. Once again, a word of caution. Birth in any sign does not indicate status. It simply points to a particular set of energies with which the individual is called on to work within a given lifetime.

The keynote of the Soul in Pisces runs: *I leave the Father's home, and turning back I save.* As we fulfil our duty in service and learn to co-operate wisely with the spiritual forces seeking to enlighten the human condition, there will come a time when we can respond to impression from depths of being even beyond the Soul. The Soul nature is an expression of Divine Love. Beyond this lies the mystery of Divine Will. The world saviour is one who is now moving on towards developing a higher sensitivity. Having developed the qualities of the Soul and generated an energy matrix as a result that rejects the separative tendency, receptivity of Divine Will becomes possible.

The world saviour makes no claim as to spiritual status. He or she knows who they are and what they are about. They have no time for guru worship, for much of this is emotionally based and generates cloud on emotional levels that threatens to obscure the light that is being carried. They would rather be allowed to continue with their work and let their radiance inspire others to discover their own field of service.

In our workshop we use a dance called White Bird, which contrasts with that used in Aries. The pattern we trace is that of a bird — head, tail and two wings. We might see it as also symbolising the dove of peace. We travel in the opposite direction, now to the right, symbolising movement into the light. The pattern of the dove is also the shape of the cross, but, whereas in Aries we sought a sense of carrying it as a burden down into the worlds of human experience, now there is a lightness. Having marked out the cross, we fly free from it, symbolising liberation. However, it is not an escape, for again and again in the dance do we mark out the same pattern, only to fly free each time. We enter the cross and all that it symbolises and yet we know we are more than what it represents. We know that we are no longer subject to its limitation as it symbolises the fourfold human personality. We are ready to take our places as conscious co-operators in the Divine process of life.

Finale

We end as we begin, once again moving in a dance around the circle in ceaseless motion, going in to the centre and returning to the circle. In the first dance, we seek to symbolise the endless chain of rebirth. Now all is different. We no longer feel subject to forces greater than ourselves, helplessly driven by human desire for experience into life after life. Now our movement is more measured and more timed. Now there is a majesty and an uprightness as we move into the centre to reach up for greater inspiration and direction. Now we move with the assurance of having realised our place and purpose in life.

Visualisation (3) — The Path of Return

The Journey into Greater Light

Sagittarius
The battles have been fought and won and a new direction is clear: the impulse now is onwards ever onwards, towards the goal of initiation. Fiery one-pointedness characterises our

striving towards spiritual sensitivity and understanding. In the dance we burned a path into the light. Impulsive? Perhaps. But there is a purpose now, the goal is seen and the will to grow urges us on towards Greater Light. The spark has sensed the flame and our face is set towards re-union. *I see the goal, I reach that goal, and then I see another.*

Capricorn

The steady perseverance of Capricorn is experienced as the goat climbs the mountain of initiation. Far more measured in our approach, we need surer footing in order to reach further towards the light. We may rest awhile on the rocky face before proceeding once more, and at times we find ourselves retracing our steps back down to undergo the experiences and lessons we need for the next phase of the ascent. There is no path behind us now, the only way is onward and upward until we reach the top of the mountain, the Light supernal that is our spiritual heritage. *Lost am I in Light supernal, yet on that Light I turn my back.*

Aquarius

Having reached the summit in Capricorn and turned, we now make our way back out into the world, drawing spirit down into matter, carrying the waters of life to thirsting humanity, showing light to the world and thereby bringing the world into the light. Our consciousness is infused with the light of the Soul, we have passed from self- to group-consciousness. We return to serve in the valley of human experience. *Water of Life am I, poured forth for thirsty men.*

Pisces

As we begin so must we return. Once more we danced the symbolic cross, yet now we fly free from it, travelling out of the dark and into the light. The four-fold personality is a trained and focused mechanism for our Soul nature to find expression in the world, an anchoring point for the energy of Will — "not my will but Thine be done". The white bird symbolises the dove of peace, and in Pisces comes the final release from the struggle of form-life and the perpetual wheel of rebirth. Not for ourselves have we undertaken this final journey though, but that we might bring liberation to others. *I leave the Father's home, and turning back I save.*

Finale

We return to the circle no longer chained to the wheel of rebirth. We have recognised the wheels within wheels of creation, and our place as individuals within them. We are now co-creators, consciously creating our own cyclic movement within the greater cyclic in-and-out breath of divinity. We move through the stages of the final dance, symbolising the zodiacal cycle, with majesty, controlled intent and spiritual purpose. We have entered Greater Light. We thereby earn the right to work in line with a Greater Will.

A Little Smackerel of Something

Richard

We have both had an interest for some while in the work of A A Milne, Lynn recalling how, when she was a teenager, her father would read the stories to himself and chortle away in his chair. I did not read the books in my early years but became more interested later in life following the publication of *The Tao of Pooh*, and hearing Alan Bennett's wonderful recordings of some of the stories on the radio.

We did not realise that we had a common interest until the first time we went away together. Lynn had decided to take her two rather ancient and very original volumes of *Winnie-the-Pooh* and *The House at Pooh Corner* with her, and announced on the first evening that she wished to read a story. Many smiles later and the response came back from me, "Can I read one now?"! It was not long before the thought emerged — how about dancing the characters?

It was in 1994 that the workshop ran for the first time and a group of avid Pooh fans assembled at Brook Village Hall in Surrey. The day included dances for each of the characters in the stories: Piglet, Owl, Kanga, Roo, Rabbit, Tigger, Eeyore, Christopher Robin and, of course, Winnie-the-Pooh. We also added a dance to represent the enchanted wood!

The thing that struck us most from the day was the depth of discussion and feeling around the personalities of the inhabitants of the Hundred Acre Wood. Everyone had their favourite, and often people found themselves defending a character that was receiving a little too much negativity from other participants. In *A Little Smackerel of Something* we always spend time brainstorming the characteristics of Pooh and his friends so that we can all get a feel for the subtle differences (and the glaringly obvious ones) among A A Milne's creations.

So let us look at each of the characters and perhaps from them learn a little about ourselves. Who shall we begin with? We begin the day with a visualisation which takes us into the Enchanted Forest. So maybe this is how we should begin now.

Visualisation to enter the Enchanted Forest

Close your eyes and imagine yourself just approaching a forest. The trees are moving gently in the breeze and as you enter them you feel a deep sense of peace pervade you. The trees are comforting, and you wander among them, touching them, communicating with them, feeling their strength and gaining nourishment from their presence.

You come across Pooh's house and who do you see with his hand in a "hunny" pot, and with "hunny" on his nose? Yes, it is Winnie-the-Pooh! He has just had a smackerel of something and is wiping the "hunny" from his face. He is about to visit his friends because it is Saturday. So he takes you by the paw and leads you to Piglet's house. Pooh knocks and slowly the door is opened by an anxious Piglet. He is timid about strange people in the forest but is very pleased to see Pooh.

The three of you set off for Owl's house. In his usual way Owl makes everything very complicated and talks far too much. He eventually decides to come along and off you all go to Rabbit's house. Rabbit is so busy doing things that he has no time to listen at first. Pooh tells him that you are all off to visit everyone because it is Saturday. Rabbit says he'll come, and insists on leading.

On the way to see Eeyore you pass Kanga's house. She is about to go and fetch Roo and Tigger who are out playing in the sand pits, so you join up with her. At the sand pit Tigger comes bouncing up to say "hello", and Roo jumps up and down squeaking "Look at me! Look at me!", and falls down a mouse-hole.

With Captain Rabbit in the lead, the happy band eventually reaches Eeyore's sad and gloomy place. He assumes you have only called on him as a last resort, or by accident. Pooh persuades him to join the party. Eeyore trudges along at the back.

Finally you all reach the top of the forest where Christopher Robin lives. You meet up with him outside his house. He is delighted to see you. "Well", says Pooh, "I think it must be time for a little smackerel of something", and you all agree. We all follow Christopher Robin into his house æ a long line of everybody.

Winnie-the-Pooh

Without doubt, Winnie-the-Pooh is more than just a bear of little brain. Throughout the stories, and regardless of the situations in which he finds himself, he discovers a way through, treading his own path through life in his own inimicable way. Nothing seems to really trouble Pooh bear. Even when there is an adventure at hand he just takes things in his stride and even when he does silly things they somehow turn out right. It is not that he does things right or wrong, but he does things his way, the Pooh way, with no malice or sinister intention. Perhaps this is why things work out for him.

We have so far used a couple of dances to represent Pooh: the first demonstrates his flowing nature, moving through life steadily towards his goal (whatever that is). The second is more reflective, revealing the thoughtful Pooh that can weigh up situations and find unexpected insight. Pooh has this wonderful non-analytical logic: he avoids worrying himself into complexity and confusion. He flows through life knowing that all will be well, and it always is.

Piglet

Well, after visiting Pooh we can be sure to find Piglet close by. Piglet is a timid creature, often quite anxious and having a habit of hopping up and down when he is unsure. Yet he has capacity to undertake courageous tasks when called upon to do so. We feel sure that within all of us there is a measure of timid Piglet. Maybe there are particular experiences that we find difficult to cope with, or situations that loom awesomely large and make us feel quite small and helpless. The Piglet personality will probably be looking for a reason to be somewhere else. Or will be looking out for a friendly paw to hold.

We human beings also like to hold a friendly paw in times of trouble and distress. We may not always admit to it. We are so conditioned in our society to be independent and self-supporting. Yet we are not all able to achieve this. We see Piglet as representing those of us who to some degree struggle with low self-esteem. We cannot quite believe in ourselves, and, even when we do the courageous act, we find ourselves wondering if it was really us, or make excuses to avoid receiving too much praise. It does not fit with our self-image. Yet the Piglets of the world can be brave, can assert themselves. They may need some encouragement and perhaps some support at first, but they can find inner strength.

In the workshop we are all given the opportunity to experience each of the characters and this is where unexpected potential can be found. People who are convinced they are one personality type discover a real feeling for, and a sense of empowerment from, another of the characters. Suddenly fresh potential is sensed. I can take the lead like Rabbit! I can bounce around in my own way like Tigger! Or maybe the dominant and assertive type discovers a gentle mothering quality as they dance into the character of Kanga.

We tend to fix our character in stone (at least in our own minds). I am a this so I cannot be or do that. How do you know? Why not try to be something a little different? Why not find out if other qualities feel natural to you and worth developing? Why not seek out other ways of being?

For Piglet we use a very bouncy dance that requires lots of little steps and a readiness to hop up and down. For those who feel they are timid Piglets the challenge is to discover the nature of their hidden strength that may be portrayed through another character. For those who deny any timidity their challenge is to accept that probably, deep down, they can be a little anxious and maybe very anxious.

Rabbit

Now Rabbit is a wonderful character, full of activity and organisation, bossing everyone around and always sure that he has the right answer, which he sometimes has, but often has not. The Rabbits of the world are the doers, the people who are only alive if they are busy, and if they cannot be busy with their own business then they will consider it their duty to busy themselves with somebody else's! We think of him as Captain Rabbit, always having to be at the front, always bustling about.

He can be frenetic, full of self-importance, pro-active and potentially thoroughly exhausting for those who get swept up and organised by him. We use a particularly fast dance that involves going from side to side and then weaving in to the centre and the net result of all our activity and movement is that we end up back where we started!

In our workshops we have all the animals in the centre of the circle, but we have searched in vain for a real Rabbit. The shops seem full of fluffy bunnies, but not the upright, imposing and, at times, extremely mischievous and vindictive Rabbit that we are seeking.

Owl

One of the delights of dancing the Winnie-the-Pooh characters lies in the contrasts. We learn much about ourselves when we dance into a character or discuss the personality type that he or she represents, but we also learn a great deal in the contrasting experience of the different characters. Owl appears wise (well he can spell Tuesday even if he doesn't spell it right) and yet he somehow never is. He uses lots of words and can be extremely philosophical, but the overwhelming feeling from the workshops is that everyone will have fallen asleep long before Owl gets to his point. He delights in words, in sharing his knowledge (which is actually rather limited) and in appearing to be the wise one.

He has one advantage over the other animals — he can fly — and in some stories this proves to be important, when messages have to be delivered, for instance. Yet with the liberation that flight brings, Owl is also extremely limited. He blusters and even when he has the knowledge, he would find it difficult to inspire others or lead them in the way that Rabbit might. Well, Rabbit would not give you any choice in the matter, you would be organised into doing what he wanted you to do and that would be that!

Owl (or Wol as he spells his name) is rather ponderous and cannot easily be knocked off his perch, literally or when he is speaking. He will carry on until he has finished. Somehow he reminds us of the absent-minded professor. The dance we use represents this ponderousness and a way of flying that is a little bit up and down, not as sure and steady as Owl might want you to think. He is a great character and I am sure that many of us find his type quite a challenge.

In our world today we see the struggle between knowledge and wisdom reflected in so many areas of human concern. Scientific knowledge has given humanity all kinds of power — some of which is real, some illusion. Power over nature is one of the illusions. Knowledge has told us we can do what we want with nature, that it will be alright. Knowledge has told us to exploit. Wisdom tells us that we must learn to listen to nature and to co-operate with her processes.

Knowledge tells us that we need a comfortable material lifestyle to be happy. Wisdom says happiness is a quality of life, not a quantity of life.

Tigger

There is no doubt that Tiggers, in any situation, are bound to make an impact on people. If their endless energy does not wear you out, you are doing well! We have found ourselves involved in discussions over the relative maturity of the Tigger type of person. On one level they can seem so insensitive and what we have termed 'self-unaware', and yet somehow we might wish for ourselves a measure of their innocence and constant enthusiasm to learn and to do.

We use a very lively and, of course, bouncy dance for Tigger so that everyone can end up feeling breathless, and often enlivened by the sheer energy of the experience. OK perhaps in short doses?

There is also something about Tigger that suggests he is not only lacking in some degree of self-consciousness; he is also often unaware of the effects he has on others. Is this insensitivity? We think not, rather, he simply lives so much in the present, in embracing the totality of his own experience with such enthusiasm, that anything beyond his immediate world of experience might as well not be there. He seems able to move from one experience to the next, not weighed down by what has happened before.

Tigger appears to be utterly fearless. It is not that he has conquered fear, he simply does not have it. His simple, yet energetic view of life has no space for fear. Tiggers, in their own minds and hearts at least, can do anything! That is until they find that they cannot do something, but this will soon be forgotten as a new experience comes along.

Eeyore

It is fascinating to contrast Tigger with Eeyore, the old grey donkey who, it seems, always likes to have a good moan. He dwells in a sad and gloomy place. Is this an outside location, or a place within himself? Yet he can be affectionate, he can be sensitive to others on occasions, but often he remains wrapped in a depressive cloud, emerging from time to time to fire sarcastic comment on the unwary.

He likes to be the centre of attention, and makes the most of it when it happens, although he would naturally assume that it was simply a mistake. He seems to be the archetypal martyr, always putting himself down, and suggesting that it is bound to rain later.

A slow plodding dance that draws us into ourselves represents Eeyore, and it really does bring us into our own sad and gloomy place. You can feel the circle contract as if each participant feels his or her individual vulnerability and seeks comfort in closeness. A real sense of introversion emerges and it was commented on one occasion how half an hour of dancing as an Eeyore would soon suck us into depression. Whilst Tigger may give us bounce, Eeyore is sure to flatten us.

Roo

In the stories, Tigger is often found playing with Roo. This seems significant, for whilst Roo is a child, Tigger is extremely childlike. Roo is always seeking excitement and attention, usually jumping up and down only to fall in a mouse hole.

There is a child in us all, and sometimes we forget this: a child that would like to play and to try to do the kinds of things that adults tell us not to do. We want to explore and experiment and to find out about things ourselves. We want to play with life but somehow it has all got far too serious and out of our control. Roo does need protecting, as we all do, from flights of fancy, but there are times when we just have to try something out for ourselves, so long as we are prepared to take responsibility or to learn from it. Adults (or our internal adult) are around to see that we do!

Roo does not know fear. He may be small, like Piglet, but he is not timid. When he is in a story he is very present and very active. The child does so like to have attention, indeed, the child needs attention as it learns who it is and where its boundaries are. Needless to say, we use a children's dance for Roo.

Kanga

Kanga is the only female in the Winnie-the-Pooh stories and stereotyped in many ways. Her role seems to be one of perpetual motherhood, protecting and nurturing Roo, and always on hand to give out his strengthening medicine. In dancing Kanga we have an opportunity to explore the gentle, caring aspect in our own natures and, in the context of the other dances, it can bring to peoples' awareness the fact that this side of human nature is more present for them than they had previously thought.

It is also intriguing to note the juxtaposition of Tigger and Kanga: Kanga, the kangaroo, you would expect to be bouncing everywhere; Tigger, the tiger, you would expect to be more steady and sure. Yet Kanga is not allowed to develop much personality in the stories, except when Piglet is substituted for Roo in her pouch and she plays along with this to maybe teach Piglet a lesson. In one workshop we found ourselves discussing how Kanga represented women and how it was tempting to say on reading the stories that Kanga is just the mother figure. To do so is to fall into a trap (and not a heffalump trap either). How dare we think of the power of nurturing and protecting as *just* motherhood. It IS motherhood and it requires to be celebrated and acknowledged as the human quality that it is.

It left us wondering what a 'politically correct' version of the stories would come out like! We decided that it would destroy them. The characters do not conform to a strong gender identity even though it is clear that all of them except Kanga are male. More important are the personalities, because they can all be found in men and women everywhere.

Kanga mothers, *in extremis* Kanga smothers. Kanga seeks to protect Roo (and Tigger) from risk. She can see a little further ahead than some of the other characters, perhaps a mother's instinct? Do not be fooled, she may not play a central role in the stories, but she is certainly a central figure in life!

Christopher Robin

In many ways Christopher Robin is the most misunderstood character within the stories. The discussions we have had reveal him to be both a little boy and, to the other animals, someone to be looked up to, almost as a saviour. He is always sought for when help is needed, with an assurance that Christopher Robin will know what to do. When there has been an adventure, and a tale to tell, it is to Christopher Robin that the animals turn. He becomes rather a confessor figure. Yet, he is still a little boy as is made so clear at the end of the stories when he has to leave the enchanted wood to go to school.

He is not really a parent to the animals, or is he? He certainly does not tell them off, but lets them have their own adventures and be themselves. He may organise them (sometimes with the assistance of Rabbit who is only too eager to oblige). Yet he himself does not always have the answer to the problems that Winnie-the-Pooh and his friends face. In fact Pooh often finds the solution and usually without realising it. We actually use a children's dance for Christopher Robin that is evocative of walking in the woods and the thrill and exhilaration of scuffing leaves with your feet — something that many children (and some adults if they let themselves) find great fun.

Christopher Robin meets the expectations of his animal friends and joins them in their play, entering into their world to share their experiences. He is accepted as he is, and he is himself, not trying to be something or somebody else.

Other activities

We include in this workshop other activities as well. The 'expotition' to find the North Pole is a favourite. It is amazing how people really get carried along by what is a very simple idea and allow a little bit of the child in them to flow freely. The location in Surrey where we have done this involved everyone having to walk past swings and a slide. Yes, nearly everyone headed over there on the way back after successfully finding the North Pole!

We also write hums, and once again it is wonderful how people really get into this. You do not have to be a poet, or an expert, to write a hum. If the words do not rhyme, well you might just make one up to get you out of trouble. One participant produced the following which we reproduce with her permission:

Hester's hum

Every day is a Happy Day
If you live your life the Poohish Way —
Look at the trees
Feel the breeze
And eat as much honey as you please.

You won't grow fat
You'll stay quite thin
If you dance in a circle with Richard and Lynn.

Dance and dance till your feet feel tired
Dance and dance and you'll feel inspired
Dance and dance till your legs feel funny
Then its time to sit down and have some more honey.

Of course, we dance the forest too, for to understand the essence of the stories we cannot just meet the characters, we have to find them in their special place. We too have our own special place. Here we can encounter those qualities realised or unrealised that are aspects of our own nature. Without doubt, this is a 'playshop', and enormous fun. A safe place to explore ourselves and to just get away from the world for a few hours. This is our "enchanted wood". We each need to find a place of enchantment. Our hectic lives, our constant urge to be busy and to struggle to keep our balance as we surf the waves of stress, keep us from finding this place. We need it, probably more than we realise …

We end with a visualisation as we depart from the enchanted wood, leaving some aspects of ourselves behind, and choosing to take newly found qualities with us back into our everyday lives.

Parting visualisation

Close your eyes and see yourself in the enchanted place in the forest sitting there seeing the whole world spread out until it reaches the sky. See each of the animals in turn come into view.

Busy Rabbit speeds past and you see how little he actually does: leave behind the need to rush, bustle and organise everyone.

Owl flies by and you see that-part-of-you-that-always-knows-best fly away with him.

Kanga is still fussing over Roo and you allow that part of you to stay in the forest.

Roo meanwhile has not grown up and you determine to remain young at heart but not childish.

Tigger is boasting about all the things he can do and you leave that aspect of you behind.

Eeyore wanders by, moaning about how badly life is treating him and you can see that only brings more sadness.

Piglet runs up to you and squeaks, "It's Today". "My favourite day" you say, vowing not to be a frightened little Piglet.

And there is Pooh. He is humming a hum which has just come to him. He flows like the water, reflects like the mirror and responds like an echo. He is a Bear of Very Little Brain but you do love him so. Pooh just is!

Just be.

You turn away to leave the forest and re-enter your everyday life.

The Cross and the Circle: Living Symbols

Lynn

It is always fascinating the way themes emerge, particularly when you are not really looking for them! I have been running alternative Christmas Days for some years and we found ourselves, after one particular Christmas, wondering whether there was scope for an alternative Easter. What form could it take? Would it attract interest?

After a good deal of thought and soul-searching we were finally struck with the obvious! What are the symbols of Easter? The cross and the circle. The cross is central to the Christian Easter experience and the circle, well, Easter Eggs for a start are sort of circular. Yet the circle is also a symbol of wholeness and completeness. It holds a promise of movement and evolution. Easter is certainly a time for moving on, for completing and beginning. Linked as it is with the full moon of Aries, the sign as we have seen of commencement, Easter marks the start of a journey. It ends with the cross and the promise of resurrection to new life and new possibilities.

This has proved to be one of our most popular workshops, bringing people some fascinating insights into the symbolism of the cross and the circle.

Easter and Easter eggs

We had a wonderful time planning our first 'Cross and Circle' day. We were surrounded by books of all sorts with pads of rough paper, making copious notes. We looked up references to these two symbols in practically every book we have — and that is a lot! We found some fascinating information. For instance, did you know that the word Easter comes from Eostre, the Saxon Goddess of Spring? Her name comes from the same root as the word oestrogen, the essence of feminine fertility. Thus Easter is inextricably linked with the idea of fertility — the 'resurrection' of spring after the 'death' of winter.

We came across many different legends about eggs. The 'cosmic egg' is the beginning of all life. In one Bronze Age Egyptian myth the egg is laid by a large goose, 'The Great Cackler', and in Greek Orphic myth the world egg is laid by uncreated night imagined as a black-winged bird. Many African and Arctic legends tell of a mythical water-bird which laid the egg of the world from which creation emerged. So the egg symbol represents the birth of the world (or the Earth) and the birth of the manifest universe.

New life cracks open the Easter egg — the ancient serpent egg laid by the Goddess, split open by the Sun God, from which each Spring the world is hatched. In neolithic times, eggs were placed on the ploughed earth to ensure the renewal of vegetation.

Interestingly we have only twice run this workshop near Easter; it is just as powerful and special at any time of year. The cross and circle are very ancient symbols, occurring in some form in most of the world's major traditions. They each have deep significance as individual symbols but also in combination, as for instance in the Celtic cross. First we investigate what they mean for us separately and then together. It seems that our workshops often fall into a threefold pattern in this way: there is a neatness about it and three is a magic number in many traditions. It represents the unmanifest becoming manifest and dividing into spirit and matter: the third element then becomes the relationship between the two. Thus we have the one becoming the two, becoming the three.

The circle

We start by considering the circle. To bring the group into the right frame of mind we do a couple of dances that emphasise this symbol. In one of them we are continually moving from two circles to one and back again. It is so simple yet it is remarkable how effective it is. In the other we move round the big circle in little circles continually changing partners and meeting new people. The dances become symbolic not only of the circle but of the cyclic nature of our lives; of cycles within cycles; of wheels within wheels.

In our experience, people find the circle a 'comfortable' symbol: it represents completeness, wholeness. There is no beginning and no end. Sitting (or dancing!) in a circle all are equal; no one person stands out from the rest as happens in a 'lecture format' of rows of chairs facing a podium.

Yet people wisely comment that the circle can also be exclusive. We seem to naturally consider it as inclusive, but that is only true for those who are actually a part of it at the time. Imagine walking into a room with a group of people already in a circle with no room for you to enter — no spare chair, or dancing in a close handhold. It is easy to feel rejected in such a situation and it is important for the existing group to consciously part company and allow in the newcomer — fetch a chair for them, open up the closed circle in some way.

The circle is traditionally a symbol of the eternal spiritual realms, the infinite, the universal and intangible. Although it is a single, self-contained unit, it encompasses everything. It is symbolic of our world, our universe and all the planets. We see the sun as circular, and the moon.

The circle also holds mystery in a mathematical sense. A circle can be drawn easily with a stick and a piece of string, yet even if we know the length of that string (the radius) we cannot calculate its circumference or its area exactly, because they are both dependent on the unresolvable fraction pi. Its dimensions thus become a reminder that the circle is infinite.

We had what we thought might be a crazy idea, to help people experience the cross and the circle. It turned out to be an extremely meaningful and powerful exercise. We get the group to just stand in those shapes! It sounds so simple yet it brings up the most amazing feelings. With eyes closed we all stand in a circle facing the centre holding hands. Then we drop hands, we turn out to face the world, we join hands again, we face round the circle — there are many different positions we can be in. We stay in each position for a while and at the end turn to the one which was most comfortable for us.

The majority will be facing the centre holding hands, but is that just the way of Circle Dancers? A few will be facing outwards: they say that they felt the strength of the circle behind them and were able to face the world with the knowledge of that backing. Some find it difficult to make a decision because each position had its plus points. After considerable discussion the group often decides that both facing in and out are necessary to balance our lives. In this way we symbolise our need for nourishment (facing in) and our need to offer ourselves out to the world (facing out). Both are important: we have to sustain ourselves as well as give to others; we have to give as well as receive. It is incredible how much insight can come from such a simple exercise.

The cross

As the circle is symbolic of the spiritual realms, so the cross is symbolic of the material world. It is often referred to as the 'cross of matter'. Yet we came across an interesting variation on this in our research. The two ends of the upright arm of the cross can represent spirit and matter; the ends of the horizontal arm masculine and feminine. In this way we see that spirit and matter have to be reconciled before masculine and feminine can be borne.

The equal-armed cross (Figure 12) is symbolic of any four equal things: the four poles, the four seasons, the four kingdoms. It is fixed, it is measurable, it is inextricably linked with the world of matter.

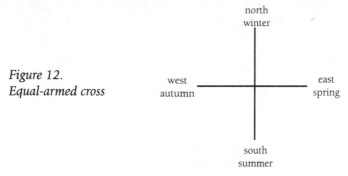

Figure 12.
Equal-armed cross

We have many familiar crosses in our lives. There is the red cross which was a symbol of true enlightenment for the Cathars and the Templars, and is now the logo and name used by one of the most caring organisations of the world. Then we have the cross of St George, which is also red on a white background. The cross of St Andrew is tilted: it is said that when he was crucified he pleaded for the cross to be in this position so that he would not die in the same way as Jesus.

This same cross has other interesting properties. It can be said to represent the combination of masculine and feminine. As shown in Figure 13, the upper part can be thought of as a chalice, the ancient symbol for the receptive feminine: the lower part becomes the sword, the equivalent symbol for the masculine. Both the sword and the chalice are necessary to make the complete cross: so too both masculine and feminine are necessary to make a complete person.

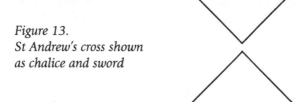

Figure 13.
St Andrew's cross shown
as chalice and sword

In the workshop we have two Circle Dances that emphasise the cross. This sounds like a contradiction but it is not. The first moves from a circle to a cross and the dancers can experience the tremendous difference in these two patterns. The second makes the shape of two crosses on the floor. It is quite an introverted dance: we are each making our own cross and it requires a certain amount of concentration on our personal movements. Yet, as somebody commented recently, when everybody was doing the movements in unison, the feeling of unity and harmony within that introversion was incredible. The quality of the dance changes when we all move together and the struggle ceases.

As with the circle, we get people to stand in the shape of a cross. They choose where they would like to be — at the top, at the bottom, on the end of an arm, or in the middle. We invite them to stand facing different directions — towards the foot of the cross or its head; all turning outwards or all inwards; sometimes they have their hands on the shoulders of the person in front, at other times they stand alone. Afterwards we ask them to return to the position which felt most uncomfortable. This varies much more than with the circle and seems to depend on where the person was standing in relation to the overall shape. There have been many insights as a result of this simple exercise.

Generally those on the ends of the arms have felt the most discomfort: it has been described as: "falling off the end"; "nobody would notice if I wasn't there". Yet someone had a wonderful sense of expanding outwards. The experience is very individual; that is why it is so powerful — we learn about ourselves.

There have been some intense reactions as well. One person described feeling quite sick when on the end of an arm and facing outwards; so much so that it was difficult to go back to that position when the instruction was given. However, when everyone was told to put their hands on the shoulders in front of them this same person felt an overwhelming sense of relief: no longer were they on their own. There was a sense of being wanted, it really felt as though they were being drawn back into the group.

At the top of the cross, there have been descriptions of a feeling of flying away. Whereas at the bottom there can be a sense of carrying the burdens of the world. In the middle there usually seems to be a sense of well-being, of being a community, of being nurtured, especially when everybody turns to the centre.

All this from just standing in a particular shape! It is not surprising then that the ancients took symbols seriously: perhaps we do too but not in quite such an open way. They can certainly give us clues as to what makes us feel comfortable or ill at ease.

The cross and the circle

When we combine these two symbols we have the idea of a moving cross. This was the symbol of the swastika which rotated anticlockwise which in our dances represents movement towards the light (the arms lead the cross into circular movement). The Nazi symbol reversed this; it thus became a rotation into the darkness. It has become a symbol of fear, yet it was originally one of hope; of the cross of matter spinning into the realm of the spiritual and the infinite (Figure 14).

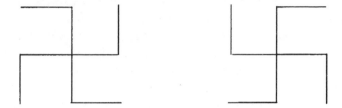

Figure 14. The original swastika rotating towards the light and the Nazi reversal

The combination of the cross and the circle can be seen in different forms in the ancient Celtic crosses and the Egyptian ankh. Isis is often depicted holding a lotus in one hand and a circle and cross (*crux ansata*) in the other. A modern use of the same symbolism is Jung's model of the life-cycle (Figure 15). In this we see our life from the point of birth, through childhood and young adulthood, to mature adulthood and finally old age, followed by death. At the pivotal point between young adulthood and mature adulthood lies mid-life — a time of crisis for many and opportunity for all.

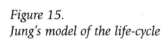

Figure 15.
Jung's model of the life-cycle

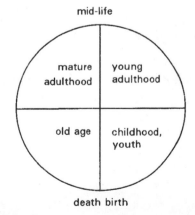

Then there is the cross and circle of the yearly cycle and the eight fire festivals. As shown in Figure 16, the solar festivals of the solstices and equinoxes can be represented as an upright cross, while the quarter days, which in our Celtic tradition were originally celebrated at full moon, can be envisaged on a tilted cross. With the advent of the Christian calendar

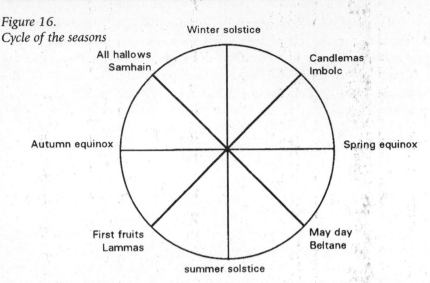

Figure 16.
Cycle of the seasons

these lunar festivals have been fixed to the first of November, February, May and August (I start with November because this was the Celtic new year). The upright cross therefore represents the masculine, solar forces, and the tilted cross the feminine, lunar aspect. As the diagram shows, we continually move between the two, changing from masculine to feminine and on again in a continuous cycle. Once again the cross and the circle are reconciled and the cycle of life is represented within the symbolism.

Let us now look at the three crosses of the cycle of the zodiac — the mutable (Gemini, Virgo, Sagittarius and Pisces), fixed (Taurus, Leo, Scorpio and Aquarius) and cardinal (Aries, Cancer, Libra and Capricorn) — as indicated in Figure 17.

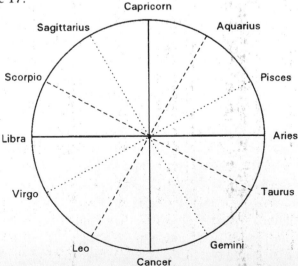

Figure 17.
Cycle of the seasons

The different crosses govern different stages on the path of conscious evolution. The mutable cross (dotted) governs normal, daily life and the growth that occurs through form experience (the cross of the hidden Christ). The fixed cross (dashed) is linked to the life of the Soul and the struggle to bring this aspect of creation into expression in matter through form (the cross of the crucified Christ). The cardinal cross (solid) is linked to the spirit and governs a further stage in human evolution that is concerned with bringing spirit into relationship with matter (the cross of the risen Christ). The three crosses correspond to Form, Soul and Spirit and together therefore correspond to a fundamental triplicity in creation.

The combination of the cross and the circle is represented by the idea of 'squaring the circle': the square being just a different style of cross. Geometrically, this involves constructing a square that has the same perimeter or the same area as the circle. We have already agreed that the relationship between the area, circumference and radius of a circle is dependent on the illusive pi, whereas the perimeter and area of a square are calculable. So the construction is necessarily approximate. Squaring the circle thus becomes an attempt to reconcile the apparent opposites of the infinity of the circle and the finite nature of the cross. Symbolically it represents the bringing of spirit down to matter. So this is the meaning of the combination of the cross and the circle.

It provides a way to help us to make sense of our lives: it seems that there is always that struggle between our material and our spiritual nature. Squaring the circle shows us that while the two can never be fully reconciled we can get very close to it. We find that symbols become doorways through which we may glimpse the truth, windows from which we can see beyond ourselves. Yet we must remember that doors can be closed and windows shuttered: they can thus serve both to reveal and conceal.

In this part of the workshop we do a number of dances which include crosses in one form or another yet move in a circular way. The cross may be marked out on the floor with the feet and the feeling is of moving from one cross to the next. In another dance we open our arms out and hold on to the next-door-but-one person and collectively our arms make a series of crosses. In this close handhold we move gently round the circle with small, neat steps. We also use a dance in which we are in a shoulder hold: here we have our hands on the shoulders of the two people next to us. In this way we each make a cross of our own body. Then the circle moves together creating the effect of a continually moving cross.

In Haiku, which is a recent choreography to a piece of music which sounds very Japanese, we are in groups of four. During the course of the dance we do not move our feet at all. Yet this is dancing, there is no doubt about it: we move our arms and create beautiful mandalas. The effect is electrifying, like a moving meditation. We start with our arms across our heart; we reach up, then round and down to the floor finally returning to the original position. We have traced a big vertical circle. We reach out to the centre of our little circle and make a cross with the other members of the group; still touching hands we move our arms out to a horizontal circle and finally back to the original position. Each group finds its own rhythm and does the dance in its own unique way. We dance the cross and the circle.

We often finish this section with a dance which has four movements that are very similar (the equal-armed cross). In the first we turn round on ourselves to the right, then we go back turning to the left; so we are making small circles within our basic four equal patterns. Then we go into the centre and back. This dance is done without holding hands and it gives a wonderful sense of personal freedom. We can express ourselves individually while still being a part of the whole. Perhaps this is the essence of the symbolism of the cross and the circle.

Visualisation

After we have discussed and danced each of the symbols we have a guided visualisation. In the one on the circle we see ourselves as surrounded by a circle of energy which interacts with the circle of our neighbour. We introduce the idea of there being, in truth, no separation: we are all interconnected; a continuum of circularity.

The cross visualisation is particularly interesting, because imagining yourself being in the shape of a cross can be quite threatening and oppressive. Yet we have had comments like "I never really understood the crucifixion until doing that visualisation". We ask people to imagine themselves as a cross with arms outstretched standing on sacred soil: in this position the heart is open. If the arms move they can create a sense of imbalance. If we look up we recognise the connection with the spiritual realms; if we look down we know the connection with the Earth. Thus we become that which connects Heaven and Earth. This is, indeed, an ancient explanation for human beings standing upright.

In the cross and circle visualisation we envision a circle of light with the shadow of a cross appearing on our body. It comes from a circular window with four panes through which light is pouring. In our visualisation we imagine ourselves passing through the window and going towards the source of the light until we become one with it. Slowly we move back and return to our original position. Is the shadow of the cross still on our body?

These visualisations have proved to be of immense value in the investigation of these ancient symbols. We learn about ourselves and how we feel as a circle, as a cross and as a combination of the two. We are in truth all of them; we are a circle of energy, we are in the shape of a cross and we are both at the same time. They give us clues as to our personality, what we are comfortable with and what we find difficult.

Sacred geometry

I have been fascinated by sacred geometry for a long time. In fact geometry was my favourite branch of mathematics at school. I guess that even then I was in some way aware of the beauty of the constructions, the irrationality of the circle and the symbolism of it all. The concepts of the infinity of the circle, the squaring of the circle, and creation of the pentagram within the circle have been used over the centuries in the architecture of sacred buildings. We decided to give a very brief introduction to these concepts in our workshop. This has proved to be a source of real insight for a number of people.

For instance, take a look at Figure 18. There you will see a circle which has been squared. An inner circle has been drawn which touches the sides of the square. It was one of those amazing moments of revelation when I heard that the ratio of the radius of the inside circle to the difference between the two radii is exactly the same as the ratio of the radius of the Earth to that of the Moon. Thus:

$$\frac{OA}{OB-OA} = \frac{\text{radius Earth}}{\text{radius Moon}}$$

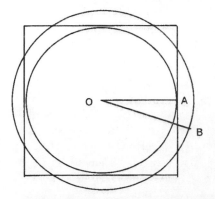

Figure 18.
Relationship between
squared circle and radii
of Earth and Moon

Artists and architects over the ages have based their work on the golden proportion. The architecture of the Parthenon in Athens, for instance, is focused on this relationship. It is basically a very simple ratio (see Figure 19). If a line AB is divided at C in such a way that the ratio AC:BC = the ratio AB:AC it is divided in the golden proportion or the golden mean.

Figure 19.
Golden proportion

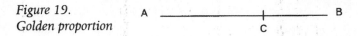

Interestingly this ratio, like pi for the circle, is not a rational number — it can be calculated to an infinite number of decimal places but never be resolved. Is it this that makes it such a pleasing proportion? Experiments have shown that people prefer rooms the length of whose walls are in this ratio. Even boxes in this same proportion are more pleasing to the eye.

Perhaps even more fascinating is that the human body is in this proportion too: the distance from the top of the head to the heart and from the heart to the feet are in the ratio of the golden mean. So too are the distances from the top of the head to the tip of the nose and the tip of the nose to the chin. Thus the human body is 'perfect' in this sense.

We then come to the Christian cross. This is based on the construction of the pentagram, which in itself is an interesting figure. The diagonals created when joining up a five-pointed star cross each other in the ratio of the golden mean. We can construct a cross with the horizontal arm part of the line joining the two points below the top of the star, and the vertical joining the top to the line between the two bottom points as shown in Figure 20.

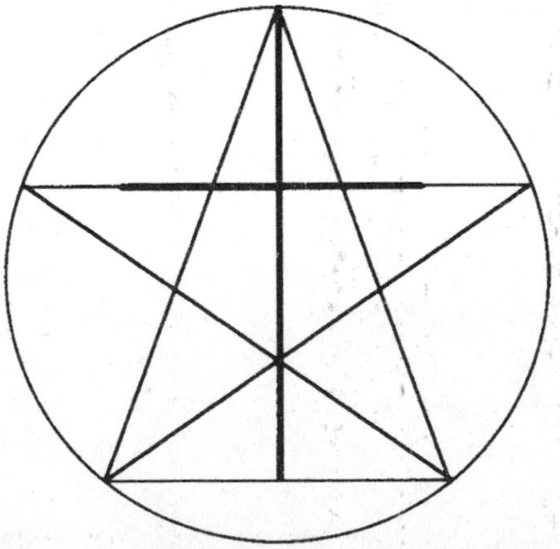

Figure 20.
Cross superimposed
on pentagram

In constructing this cross I have made the horizontal arm equal to the bottom part of the vertical arm. An optical illusion is created here: to the naked eye it looks as though the horizontal arm is much shorter. Because of the properties of the pentagram the horizontal arm of this cross cuts the vertical in the ratio of the golden mean. Thus the two arms of the cross are also in that ratio.

Recently we came across an interesting explanation of why people were crucified in many cultures. The golden mean was considered the perfect proportion and, as we have seen Man is created in that ratio. The crucifixion, then, was not so much a matter of punishment for crime committed as an attempt to help the criminal conform to the ideal, to become one with the true inner being.

We have found that sacred geometry is a new topic for many people and they express surprise and wonder at the aspects we have chosen to highlight. Often they go away fired with enthusiasm and intent on pursuing their own investigation. This is, after all, of necessity only a brief encounter with the rich realms of a subject as old as building itself. It explains the thinking behind the architecture of many of our best loved old buildings — cathedrals and churches, as you might expect, are designed along these lines. It is a huge subject into which we can only dip our toes in such a short time.

Mandalas

So now it is time for tea! But we have another surprise in store for our guests. We make the tea — although that is not the surprise! — while they are given the opportunity to create their own mandala based on the cross and the circle. They each have an A3 sheet of paper which has an outline of a circle drawn on it. There are rulers, crayons, coloured pens, wax crayons and chalks. The choice is theirs as to how to create their picture. What it represents is also up to the individual: it might be the person's own life-cycle, the cycle of the seasons or simply a beautiful picture in circular form.

We have had a range of responses to this idea. "I can't draw." "How wonderful to be able to express myself in colour." "I'm not an artist." "This is the best part of the day." We have had those who refuse point blank to do it! Well, that is alright with us: we are not going to force anyone. On one occasion one such person, who said she could not draw, was seen after about two minutes to take a piece of paper, some crayons and hide herself in the corner. She came back with an amazingly beautiful pattern of colour, immediately putting the lie to her statement that she could not do it.

This exercise has produced some lovely results. One person drew a tree with branches reaching into each segment. As she explained, "This represents my growth in life, the stability of my roots in the ground, and reaching up to the sky and to something beyond". Another participant was aiming to "just put colour on paper with no clear intention of what it represented". As she said after the allotted 15 minutes, "I keep seeing more and more in it".

I am no artist — I was told that at school and have resolutely believed it ever since. Yet the very act of putting colour on paper is creative: it does not have to be a Rembrandt or Picasso. That is not the objective. The essence of it is to express ourselves in our own unique way, to create something of ourselves, for ourselves. Most people do not want to share their efforts: that is fine. It is, after all, a very personal experience and whatever you create is part of you. To share it may detract from it. We have certainly witnessed over a number of workshops what a powerful experience it can be to produce your own mandala.

So to completion

We are nearly at the end of the day. It remains to clear up the colouring tools, give people a last opportunity to share anything they want to, and do one more dance. We do a thanksgiving dance in which we reach down to the floor, metaphorically picking up whatever we choose, bring it to our heart centre with arms crossed, and then offer it up in thanksgiving, opening our arms and heart wide, finally bringing our arms down in a circular movement and joining hands ready to move on. Again we make the symbols of the cross and the circle: we emphasise in this last dance the whole meaning of the day.

We finish with a Buddhist blessing (The Blessing of the Four Divine States) to the four corners of the world: by now we are familiar with the symbolic aspect of this final ritual. We are ready to rejoin the outside world, having shared a day which we hope has given new insights to those who have joined us.

Love to all Beings
North – South
East – West
Above – Below
Love to all Beings

Compassion to all Beings
North – South
East – West
Above – Below
Compassion to all Beings

Joy to all Beings
North – South
East – West
Above – Below
Joy to all Beings

Serenity to all Beings
North – South
East – West
Above – Below
Serenity to all Beings

Beyond Balance — Towards Complementarity

Lynn

I had been reading a wonderful book called *The Myth of the Goddess* by Anne Baring and Jules Cashford.[18] Towards the end is a chapter entitled "The Sacred Marriage of Goddess and God", which I found inspiring. It is about the interrelation of masculine and feminine. At one point the significance of the yin yang symbol (Figure 21) is described — the movement of the whole symbol and the fact that it is not divided straight down the middle so that the distinction between yin and yang is not absolute. Also,

18 .   Anne Baring and Jules Cashford, *The Myth of the Goddess: Evolution of an Image* (Viking Arkana, London, 1991).

Figure 21.
Yin yang symbol

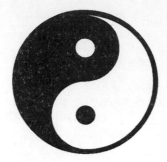

within the yin is a dot that is the essence of yang and vice versa. Both aspects are absolutely necessary to create the overall picture that we know so well.

The authors suggest that this symbol encourages us to see yin and yang not so much as opposites but as complements. When I read this sentence I was so excited I could not wait for Richard to come home. I immediately saw a new workshop forming. The concept that we should not be trying to balance opposites but considering them as complements seems to me to extend way beyond the picture of yin yang. This could be applied to so many things in our lives.

We are often exhorted to maintain a balance. Yet, if that is what we are doing, the imagery leads us to think that we are continually walking a tightrope or sitting at the fulcrum of a see-saw trying desperately to keep both ends off the ground. We are wavering from one extreme to the other and never actually achieving anything. If two things are opposites they are in continual conflict; if they are complementary they are both necessary to make up the whole. How much more positive this becomes: no longer do we have positive and negative, good and bad. Both these concepts can be transcended once we acknowledge the need for both aspects in our lives.

As with so many of our workshops we found that these concepts fell neatly into a triplicity: first we look at pairs of what we are conditioned to consider as opposites; then we imagine them as complements and feel the difference this makes; finally we draw them together so that the polarity can be transcended.

Opposites

We really involve the whole group in our workshops so that they can experience some of the creativity of making the day for themselves, both individually and as a group. So the first activity is to make a list of characteristics that are normally referred to as opposites. This usually involves Richard writing as fast as he can on the flip-chart to try to keep up with the barrage of pairs. Is it any wonder that we think so much in terms of black and white when we are surrounded by this negative way of thinking all the time?

The list will include young and old; good and bad; male and female; left and right; war and peace. In fact I guess it could go on for ever, so we have to restrict the time we have. It is a salutary exercise though to see how long the list becomes in only ten minutes.

From this sheet of paper we pick a few to dance. We have a warrior dance from Macedonia which is very energetic with a lot of stamps, followed by a peace dance from Israel which is gentle, quiet and caring. We have a men's version of a Macedonian dance called Pravo Oro which is powerful, centred and exhibitionist: it is in sharp contrast to the women's version which is done in a close handhold, to a beautiful piece of unaccompanied singing by a group of women. Interestingly the two dances have very similar steps, the men's dance moving to the right and ending with a lift to either side, and the women's dance moving to the left with a point to left and right at the end. Yet the difference between the two is enormous in terms of the atmosphere that they create.

Dark and light will usually feature on our list and we have a strong, fast and direct dance from Thrace in Greece to represent the Sun: we make the rays as we move out from the circle, then we step back to the middle, finally moving round the centre making the body of the Sun, and preparing ourselves for the next raying out of sunlight. The Moon dance that is its pair is to a beautiful adagio by Vivaldi and we trace the pattern of a crescent moon on the floor, gradually moving round the circle making the full moon. Both these dances are done in open circles with close handholds but the first leaves us a little breathless, while the second brings repose. It is so like day and night — we need the darkness to relax before the rigours of the next day. We already feel the necessity to recognise both of the pair of opposites.

If fire and water have been mentioned as opposites we do a fire dance which is fast, full of leaps and arm movements representing flames, and ends with a resounding stamp. In the 'water' dance we sway gently and rhythmically backwards and forwards, then move with tiny steps to the right in a lovely flowing sequence. The contrast again is incredible.

It is wonderful to do these dances with this intention of bringing out the contrasts, the opposites. It really emphasises the polarity that we are considering. In our everyday life these attributes are always with us: it seems that we are encouraged to look at them in terms of opposites and this brings with it an aspect of judgement.

We have devised a visualisation that emphasises this concept of polarity with which we are all so familiar. In it we look at a part of our life which we feel is out of balance. We focus initially on the quality that *is* there and then shift it towards the 'opposite' quality. We see the value of this other aspect and determine how to bring it into our life. Finally we imagine how we might act now with this fresh quality within our personality.

In the discussion after this visualisation it is surprising what has come up for people and how determined they are to make changes as a result of it. The dances, visualisation and group interaction have enabled them to reassess their lives and see new ways of acting and reacting.

Complements

So how can we rethink our world of duality? In small groups we discuss the possibility of considering the opposites as complements. Does this make us feel different? Does it change our perception of the 'opposite' qualities? What we have found is that with this new approach people feel much more positive. Life is no longer a balancing act with us perched in the middle trying not to let one side outweigh the other. We can now allow both to co-exist; we can encompass and enjoy both. Both darkness and light are essential: it is unrealistic to think that all can be light. In fact there would be no light without darkness because it would have no meaning. The two are both necessary: to label one positive and the other negative is counter-productive.

This changes the way we perceive reality. The mind naturally seeks to separate, to divide, and a dualistic world ensues. Yet when we try to isolate one pole, the other automatically appears because they are inseparable, bound together in a form of unity. One cannot exist without the other.

Here we are experiencing this powerful concept of opposites becoming complements which is so much a part of the ancient philosophy of the Gods and Goddesses. We have Kali who was the healer and the bringer of illness; the creator and the destroyer. Shiva too had these two elements of creation and destruction in harmony. Artemis was the slayer of the deer and the holder of the torch: she thus represented both dark and light. Here we have, in different traditions, an acknowledgement of the necessity of both poles and a representation of the concept of complementarity. Indeed, only by experiencing the fragments, and perhaps more importantly their relationship with each other, can we fully experience the whole.

At one workshop somebody pointed out that usually we perceive the opposites as being in a straight line with one at each end (Figure 22). This gives rise to the idea of a see-saw and living a precarious life struggling to maintain balance. If we think again we may see that often what happens is that the two poles are moving round a circle and meeting at the other end. One pole becomes indistinguishable from the other.

Consider the situation in Russia at the beginning of the century. The Revolution took the people out of a very oppressive regime controlled by the far right in the form of the Tsars. It was replaced by the far-left Communist era which proved to be no less repressive. The two poles had 'come full circle' — we even have the expression in our colloquial language. Both extremes became totalitarian: this is the danger when any opposite dominates *in extremis* — it rules out alternatives and choice, and diminishes the individual potential for creative expression.

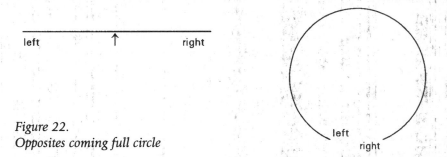

Figure 22.
Opposites coming full circle

Have you ever thought how curious it is that 'opposites' can generate similar effects? For instance, both intense heat and intense cold can burn. Extreme darkness and extreme light are blinding to the human eye. So we have the same effect, different cause — indeed the causes are literally poles apart. Returning to Figure 22 we see that the position furthest away from the effects of the extreme poles is at the high point of the circle above the extremes — the point of freedom. We shall come back to this concept in a slightly different form later in this chapter.

So we have the concept of complements and we do a number of dances that demonstrate the idea of the two poles being necessary to make up the whole. There is one that always makes a big impression: it tells the story of an old woman whose joints are becoming stiff and painful: she cannot move quite like she used to. She dances sedately, slightly ponderously; then she remembers her youth and, while dancing exactly the same steps, she leaps round the room, with great energy and excitement. The two aspects are absolutely essential to provide the mood and experience of the dance. What I find fascinating about it is that she ends up as the young woman; it is as if acknowledging that both parts of her still exist has changed her view of her current life, maybe not physically but at least mentally.

Another great favourite in this part of the workshop is a Greek dance which is all about different aspects of opening and closing. There are four sequences of three steps: in the first we move forward; in the second we turn round and move backwards with our hands held high opening right up; in the third we move forward again; and in the fourth we bend forward closing right down — even the steps are about closing as we go forward, back and together. The opening and closing are both essential elements to make the complete dance. Yet it does not stop there. While continuing in this pattern of steps we move in a spiral towards the centre — another aspect of closing. We go down into the darkness as we spiral in: on reaching the centre we retrace our steps, moving between the lines of people going in, and open back out again into the light.

The essence of this dance is that it is necessary to both open and close at different times in our lives. We have to move down into the darkness in the depths at the centre of the spiral and let go of (or sacrifice) what we no longer require: then we are free to emerge again into the light. We can then take *our* light out in to the world.

We have a number of images which we use here. What happens when others deny one pole of our nature? Usually it is the dark side which is not acknowledged and we have the 'pedestal complex'. It is very hard to live standing on a pedestal all the time. One false move and we have fallen off; then we are no longer seen as 'wonderful' and 'marvellous' but as 'awful' and 'cruel'. Yet in truth we are only human with our very human faults, or should I say with our glorious array of complementary aspects. Another feature of this is that people can assume the pedestal position and from it attempt to maintain power over others: a kind of 'cult complex' emerges and followers suppress their own power leaving them vulnerable to exploitation.

We also have the concept of the scapegoat. In this situation, faults, real or imagined, are projected onto one person. This can happen to the extent that the 'victim' believes them to be real and may begin living up (or down) to them.

Another idea which seems to ring bells for people is that of the magnet. In us, all opposites are united through the heart: we can think of this as symbolised in the magnet, which can only function when its 'opposites' are brought into relationship. Positive and negative are both absolutely essential before it can operate. If we seek only pleasure and deny/repel pain, we do not establish a tension of the opposites. We lock ourselves into our desires which are rooted in the activity of the solar plexus centre. When we hold the opposites as complements, we create a point of tension that induces the opening of the heart and the possibility of movement beyond their limiting effect. It is not that we have sought to escape from the opposites (which is an act of desire) but rather that we embrace both.

Transcending the opposites

So we have investigated the idea of opposites and introduced the concept of complements. We have another treat in store as we suggest that we can actually transcend the opposites. Consider again our straight line image with left and right on either end (Figure 22). We are only thinking in one-dimension in this picture: even if we believe that left and right are both necessary we are still standing at the fulcrum trying to accept both in our lives — we can only look at one end of the line at once.

Consider now the idea of standing above the line and introducing a second dimension to the image. At a point above the middle of the line we can see both ends; we can truly bring the two aspects into a complementary relationship. To illustrate this we have a miniature pair of scales which is pivoted above the two pans. From that point — a single point — we can observe both poles and resolve the differences between the two. We see this as a triangle (Figure 23).

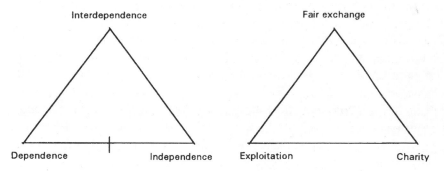

Figure 23. Triangle resolving opposites

In the figure is an example of what we are trying to convey. In fact the two triangles illustrated can be considered to be the same, with different words representing the concepts. We have a number of other triplicities like this to set people thinking how they can resolve their own pairs of opposites. It is as if we can gradually bring the two outer points of our original line closer together by rising above them and moving to this higher point of recognition, acceptance and resolution. In small groups we discuss the process of resolving various of the original pairs from our list at the beginning of the day.

In the left-hand diagram of Figure 23 there is a line in the centre of the two original 'opposites'. This is the point of balance that we are so often exhorted to find; the point of compromise. It can be an uncomfortable position in which we do not relate to either of the two qualities. The point of transcendence at the apex of the triangle is a comfortable place where the 'opposites' have come together and live in harmony.

Now we have a triangle — a two-dimensional figure. In our workshop we extend this image further. We have a cardboard circle which lies flat on the floor: however, it has been cut into a spiral and, when it is lifted from the centre, it takes on three-dimensional form. We then see that we can move continuously round the circumference going slowly up the rings of the spiral until we reach the high point, from which we are able to truly rejoice in the existence of the two aspects we had previously thought of as 'good' and 'bad'.

These two qualities of good and bad came up the first time we ran this workshop. They are a well-known pair of opposites and as a group we realised that the centre point of the line between them represents a nothingness, almost a point of apathy, where neither good nor bad can exist. The transcendent point at the top of the triangle is 'the best I can'. It is a point of power, because it is non-judgmental: it is neither good nor bad but the best that is possible — and who can complain about that? It is the 'point of freedom' which I previously mentioned in relation to the open circle in Figure 22.

After discussing the use of this image of the triangle to rise above the 'opposites' and make them truly into 'complements', we lead the group in a meditation in which we visualise ourselves as the set of scales, with one of a pair of opposites in each dish. We attempt to bring the scales into balance from that point above: we recognise that the two pans represent parts of a greater quality which combines the two, that transcends them both. From this vantage point, we acknowledge the presence of the opposites yet are free of their dominance.

This has proved to be a very revealing exercise. The imagery is so simple, yet some people find themselves struggling to attain that balance between their pans: this tells them about something that they can work with in their lives to help them to bring their two aspects into co-operation. Others find to their amazement that their two pans are already in harmony: again this is an indication of how those parts of their lives are working well together. Why not try it for yourself?

Dancing the resolution

The dance we use to demonstrate this idea of transcending the opposites is very unusual and I suppose not strictly a circle dance at all. It is called the Yin Yang dance, so despite its nature it is highly appropriate. Two people take on the roles of Sun and Moon: the Sun stands with arms wide open above the head, while the Moon has the hands crossed in front of the heart and the body slightly bowed. Here we have the complementary aspects of the opening, light and brazen Sun, with the closing, dark and submissive Moon. The other participants form short lines and move using a very simple 'forward, touch' step round the room. As a line moves between the Sun and Moon, the two people slowly swap roles — the Sun becomes the Moon, and the Moon the Sun. So we are representing the transcendence of the two extremes, one changing into the other slowly and effortlessly.

The music lasts for about twenty minutes, much longer than our usual dances: it gives time to create an atmosphere of meditation and deep peace. As a group we seem to transcend our dualistic world and become one even though we all have different roles. It is a powerful and very moving dance: it is simple and yet dramatic. The two people who are the Sun and the Moon are often particularly struck by the effect on them. They have formed a bond in the dance: they are two parts of the same entity, one becoming the other in continuous rotation.

The dance is so gentle, so slow and yet it shows us very poignantly that we are able to rise above the 'opposites' that are so familiar. We can move between them and change them one into the other. No more teetering at that precarious point of balance: we now have a much more stable point from which to view the world. It is a point that honours both aspects and seeks to bring them into harmony and wholeness.

Closing and blessing

People go away from this workshop with much to think about. The ideas we have explored give them a new way of looking at the conflicting qualities and aspects of their lives. There is ample scope for investigating this further and working on transcending the opposites in each of our characters: we can consider how to resolve the occasions when we feel pulled in two different directions. We now have a mental picture of how we might do this: we stand above the situation and bring the two pans of the scales into balance.

We have discovered how strong the tendency is to think in terms of

opposites: we have also found that it is liberating to reconsider these as complements — there is a peacefulness about the idea that both can and must co-exist and we have to bring them together in harmony.
I leave you with one more triangle to think about.

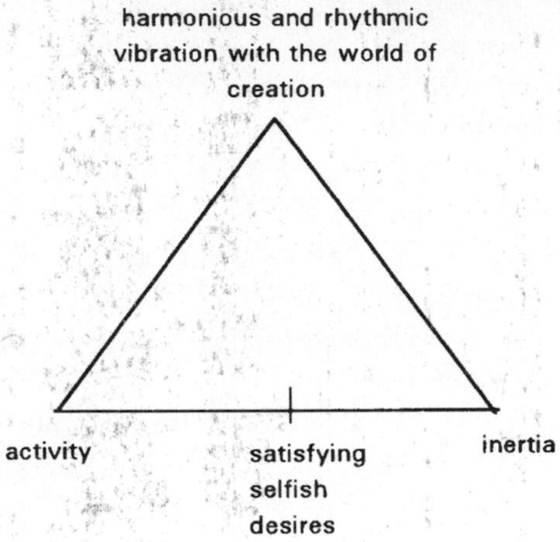

Figure 24.
Living harmoniously

harmonious and rhythmic
vibration with the world of
creation

activity   satisfying   inertia
                    selfish
                    desires

Celebrating the Spirit in a Material World

Lynn

Over a period of about ten years I have been involved in running seven or eight alternative Christmas days. The idea germinated when I realised that I no longer wanted the sort of Christmas that I was used to. I found then that many other people felt similarly. It started with a 'one-off', an experiment to see how it might work. It grew and became something of an institution, with some folk depending on it to solve their Christmas dilemma — should I go to ...? have I the courage to do what I want to and stay at home on my own? It seems as though Christmas is a time of 'shoulds' and 'oughts', of expectations by others, of others, and even thinking we know what others want us to do.

I decided that I wanted to offer an opportunity for people to explore Christmas in a new way. The days were full of love and caring. Everyone contributed. At the very start we decided what we were going to do: this usually included some time set aside to discuss the significance of Christmas and what it meant for us individually; there was usually a walk after lunch, except the year when it poured with rain; we danced; we sang; some people brought items they wanted to read to the group; we even played games; and generally we had a wonderful time.

I know many women who feel tied to the kitchen at Christmas: this is still true despite the idea of liberation. So for many of them I guess the highlight was the incredible banquet that appeared at lunchtime, each person having brought a contribution towards a shared meal — and the men provided anything from cakes they had made themselves to cheesy jacket potatoes. The washing up, too, was shared, making the whole experience of the meal one in which everyone participated.

There came a time when I felt that I needed a change from this type of Christmas and I took myself off to Nepal! It seems a bit extreme but it was a truly enlightening experience and comes thoroughly recommended as a way to get away from the glitz and glamour of Christmas. That, however, is not part of the subject matter of this book.

Another few Christmases passed by with an alternative day or two and then Richard and I decided to run a pre-Christmas workshop. The first one was on 2 December so was close to the start of Advent, the beginning of the Christmas period in the Church calendar. For me this is a time in the cycle of the seasons when we are still going down into darkness, a time for inner reflection and renewal. The frenetic shopping for presents and the panic I witness these days is far removed from the original festival of Christmas which celebrated the first day when the sun stayed out longer — the birth of the Sun or Son.

So 'Celebrating the Spirit in a Material World' was born out of this backdrop of wanting to acknowledge Christmas in my own way. It is hard sometimes to stand back from the lure of the lights and lasciviousness: we intended to provide a space to do this and to look at how we might live a spiritual life within the framework of our modern materialistic world (and at a time of year when material wants rather than spiritual needs seem to be uppermost in most people's minds).

About a fortnight beforehand we went out for a walk one Sunday afternoon. It was cold and crisp and seemed to clear all the cobwebs and leave us open and free to accept whatever flowed. We had no intention of planning the workshop when we left home, but an hour and a half later we arrived back with not just an outline of the day but a good idea of the dances we were going to use as well. This often happens to us: we rarely sit down and plan a day step by step; it is much more likely that an unexpected remark will set us both thinking, or we will be doing something totally different and a spark of an idea comes to the surface and the creative process is kindled. Do we have the ideas, or do the ideas have us?

So the framework was there and once again it fell into three phases: first we would look at the divine and its cyclic emergence — the presence of the Spirit in the world; then we would look at the concept of group unity, and Spirit in the group context; finally we would come to the personal and how we actually live the Spirit as individuals. Interestingly, our workshops often take the overall format of first looking at the particular, and gradually expanding that out to the universal or general. This is perhaps an obvious approach, because we can identify with our own experience and then it is easier to take that into a world view. In this instance though it seemed important to acknowledge the presence of Spirit universally and then bring it down first into our collective then our individual lives. This seems particularly pertinent as we move towards Aquarius and a greater seventh Ray influence which tends to promote the drawing down of spirit into matter.

Divine presence

At the beginning of each workshop we like to do one dance before introductions. The power of the dance is its ability to bring disparate people together in a harmony which is not dependent on knowing anything about the other members of the group, not even their names. In this workshop, we begin with a dance which we knew we wanted to include in the day even if it was just for its title — Song of the Soul. When we were planning the dances we had trouble fitting this one into one of our three categories: then the light dawned — it could fit in any or all, so let us use it as a common theme throughout the day.

Paradox

It is a dance choreographed to a song by Chris Williamson on the album "The Changer and the Changed". The words are a powerful acknowledgement of the presence of a Divine Spirit within our lives. It is about living with the certainty that there is something greater, a guiding light both beyond and within us. This is a wonderful paradox: the idea that divinity is both outside and inside us. Yet that is how I perceive it. If I let go of trying to understand it, I know it. It defies logic so leave logic behind and enter into a deeper way of knowing.

I love paradox; it has always fascinated me. It is a puzzle that I can only solve if I stop trying to think about it and just let it be. Maybe that is the essence of life. There is a beautiful piece in the *Book of the Runes* about living "an ordinary life in a non-ordinary way". What a paradox, yet I know the wisdom of it. We are part of the world and so we must live an 'ordinary' life; yet we are also spirit with that spark of divinity, so, to acknowledge that is to live in a 'non-ordinary' way.

Another one I like is the idea of 'purposeful spontaneity': this is an expression I first heard from a very dear and wise friend of ours. The two concepts seem to be contradictory but there is sense in the phrase. Yes, be spontaneous, and let it have a purpose. Let our lives be joyful and flowing, allowing the unexpected to take its place, and underlying that let us have a clear idea of our deeper connection and a sense of direction towards a higher goal.

Perfection is a notion that I find fascinating, because that too leads to a paradox. We may strive to be perfect yet by our very nature as human beings that is probably impossible. For a moment let us assume that somebody was perfect. I think they would be very difficult to live with, or even communicate with, so are they really perfect? Or am I confusing perfection with the old saying "I used to be conceited: now I am perfect!"? What is perfection anyway? Perhaps there is a sense in which we are 'perfect' as we are with all our 'imperfections'.

Back to Song of the Soul. We use this dance again and again throughout the day: by revisiting a dance in this way we reinforce the experience and it becomes familiar. The more familiar a dance is the more we can 'sink into' it, and it takes on a different dimension. We find new meaning in the movements if we no longer have to think about where to put our feet next. We start to 'be danced' instead of the head interfering and telling us what to do.

Cyclical emergence of spirit

In this first section we investigate the essential divinity of all things and venerate the reality of spirit in our lives from different points of view. We look at the cyclical emergence of spirit: we witness this in Nature in the cycle of the seasons but it is just as true for us. We recognise the divine presence more consciously at some times than others. Yet we ask people to consider: is it divinity that has a cyclical nature or our identification with it? In a sense it is both. Whilst spiritual impulse cyclically reaches towards the consciousness of humanity, we set aside time ourselves to cyclically engage with the spirit.

In many religions there are particular times of day, of the week or of the year set aside for prayer or celebration of the Divine presence. Many people see the full moon as a time of opportunity, when spiritual energies are more than usually available. Groups and individuals make a point of meditating at this time to tune into the cycle. So there is both a reaching up and a reaching down in synchronicity. The Divine is constant and ever-present, yet we can feel its presence more at some times than others.

We recognise a number of different time cycles from the daily meditation, through the monthly full moon, to a much bigger one governing the appearance of visionaries with new ideas in all areas of human expression. We see in this the familiar idea of cycles within cycles, wheels within wheels, of the 'micro' within the 'macro' — and even "as above so below".

Dancing the spirit

Gabrielle Wosien has choreographed a dance in the Indian tradition to a beautiful song called Jane Log (pronounced 'Jannay Log'). The whole sequence is done without joining hands. We start with our hands in the 'namaste' or prayer position. In India this is the usual greeting: it means 'I acknowledge the divinity within you'. What a lovely way to say 'hello'. When I was in Nepal wherever we went the people came rushing across the fields to greet us with namaste: in this way the spiritual came first although it was usually followed by very material requests like "Gimme-one-pen" — yes it is all one word to the children in Nepal, as is "Hellogoodbye"!

Jane Log goes on to represent Shiva in two aspects: destruction and creation. Eastern philosophy acknowledges the essential duality of the world — we have to destroy in order to create, we have to let go of the old before something new can enter our lives. Nature shows us this clearly with the leaves falling from the trees in the autumn, providing compost for the roots and allowing the new growth to appear in the spring.

So in this part of the dance we recognise the Divine in the form of Shiva: we stand on one leg throughout the slow arm movements. Some people find this quite difficult and start to question whether the balance has gone out of their lives. We are often so busy with our jobs, family and friends that we do not stop to consider the spiritual aspect. Even at a purely physical level the difficulty of standing on one leg is interesting. In my experience it is frequently an indication of having little bodily aware- ness, of not being sure where the centre of gravity is, and even of believing that it is hard to do. This last is probably the overriding factor. The mind is extremely powerful. If I believe I cannot, I probably will not! So there are a number of lessons from this simple, slow movement of the arms.

Next we become the disciple. We cross our hands across our heart and walk round in a small circle to the right. Then we reverse the turn and open our hands out wide. We are representing the path of the devotee in taking love into his/her own heart before giving it out to the world. How important this is: we cannot expect to give love to others unless we have experienced it and made it a part of our lives. We have to receive in order to be able to give.

In the final part we go to the temple carrying our candle, our light, with us in dedication. The left hand makes the dish on which the candle, the right hand, sits and the flame, the fingers of the right hand, flickers. So in the course of the dance we recognise the presence of the Divine, we represent our journey as devotees and we take our light into the temple of life. The sequence of these patterns is interesting: as the dance progresses, we no longer go to the temple, but do an extra 'devotee': it is as if the temple becomes internal as we gain more spiritual insight.

The second dance involves turning round on ourselves to the right, back to the left, into the centre lifting our arms up high in aspiration, and then coming out to start again. Four simple movements of three steps each, but what power they hold. Some people find their hands tingling as if they have been charged with energy. One person had a tremendous feeling of personal power: he is tall and quite broad. "I often feel some- what restricted in Circle Dancing because of the size of those around me," he explained. "I'm usually afraid to express myself fully in case I dominate others. In that dance I was free to find myself and be myself." He was recognising the power of that freedom. It represents the univer- sality, the vastness and the space of the Divine as well as its cyclic process.

We were amazed when we first planned this workshop to find that the first three dances were done as individuals, although the bulk of my repertoire is in a closed circle. We are continually surprised at how these workshops develop: a theme will be apparent without our introducing it consciously. Yet when we think about it we realise what is taking place. In this instance it seems that it is symbolic of us each having to find our own spirituality in our own way. We may be part of a group, yet it is still an individual journey: nobody else can travel the road for us. We may learn from others yet it is only when we take it on board for ourselves that it has any meaning for us. We have to acknowledge our own spirituality in our own hearts.

For us as facilitators the whole process is one of personal growth. We learn at least as much from planning these events as do the participants in them. It is a remarkable experience and we feel very privileged to have found such a wonderful way of discovering new insights about ourselves and the philosophy of life, and being able to share it with others. Perhaps we are back to the devotee in Jane Log who has to take the lesson, the light, into their own heart before giving out to the world. The insights seem to be all the more powerful too because they are our own: nobody has told us, we have found out for ourselves. The whole process reinforces our purpose in running the workshops — to throw out threads of light, seed thoughts for others to grasp if they will and use in their own way. We are encouraging others to find *their* own truth by direct experience, not feeding information to a passive audience.

This is the essence of 'purposeful spontaneity': we carry a purpose into our planning but the actual creativity and expression has a quality of spontaneity. We purposely create a space in which to work, yet we often find ourselves adjusting the content to suit the situation and the needs of the participants. We have sometimes reduced dramatically the number of dances we use; on other occasions we have left out part of our original programme because the discussion around what we had already done was so important and was sparking off such helpful responses. The space we work with, or the framework we create, aims to generate containment rather than constraint and frees us and the rest of the group to take risks and to explore experiences.

The third dance is representative of this process. In the movements we first look at ourselves as if reflected in a mirror and then, with a hop and a flourish, offer out to the world in joy, excitement and vitality. We return then to our own inner journey. This is important to remember: we have to nourish ourselves as well as giving out to others. It is not selfish; it is vital. On one occasion Richard was struck by the significance of the hop in the context of the theme of the workshop. It seemed to reflect our need to time ourselves before moving forward in life. If we get the timing of the hop right we are ready to move on and all runs smoothly; if we are late, we are left one step behind. There is no time for procrastination — the energy touches and inspires action and movement. The hop prepares us, symbolising our response to our inflow of energy, and then we move on, carrying it into expression in line with an inner rhythm.

We chose the last dance in the investigation of the Divine presence because of the simplicity of the footwork and the continuous motion of the arms; as soon as they reach one position they move on to the next. In the context of this workshop we recognise the simplicity of spirit, its continual, immutable presence. Richard has coined a phrase, the "on-and-onness" of spirit, which seems to capture the feeling we are trying to engender. Interestingly, in our notes we found that he had typed this as "on-and-oneness", which is perhaps even closer to the truth!

After doing these dances there is generally a sense of upliftment, of connection with our spiritual natures and the very essence of ourselves. An atmosphere of calm pervades the room and the circle: "This is how I would like to feel always". The dances seem to bring a certainty about the presence of the Divine spark within us all, and in this knowledge we experience an 'at-onement'. For we are one, each a different expression of the one truth.

In the meditation that follows we each imagine a symbol which for us represents divinity and reflect on the essence of this image. We consider how we can carry this essence of divinity into our individual sphere of influence in the world in a practical way. This is a service to humanity and must be rooted in practical application. The whole idea of the day is to look at how we can live a spiritual life in this intensely material world. We conclude with the "Affirmation of the Disciple"[19] with its wonderful first line "I am a point of light within a greater light". This in itself is enough to meditate on: for me it confirms my connection with the Divine and thus with all humanity. We are all one.

Spirit in the group

Sharing food

Lunch provides an opportunity to experience the group in a very special way. We all bring food to share and, without any planning, a wonderful spread appears. It always fascinates me to see dish after dish being placed

---

19. Copies of " The Affirmation of the Disciple" are available from World Goodwill, Suite 54, 3 Whitehall Court, London SW1A 2EF.

in the centre of the circle. There is a rich variety of food and nothing is duplicated. Those who are unused to shared food think they have to organise it to avoid having all salads or all quiches, but it never happens that way. Even in a small group the contributions are all different: we just have to trust that it will work out right. Sharing food is a beautiful expression of the idea of spirit in the group: we all prepare the food with love; we all appreciate each other's effort; and we are sustained and nourished by the food and the presentation of it. And of course we share in the chores as well, by clearing up and washing up. The whole process becomes one of group interweaving and co-operation.

The sharing of food is a powerful symbol of community. It can bring families together, and enable cultures to meet in a spirit of fellowship. In a world in which so many starve daily there is a need to remember the significance of sharing food and nourishment, and the consequences when we do not.

Common purpose

So to the dance. In this part of the day we focus on uniting the group in a common purpose, while acknowledging and celebrating the diversity of ability and character. We are looking at group relationship.

We start with a dance in a close front basket-weave handhold. Moving in such a close position we have to co-operate: we must all take small steps otherwise we would tread on our neighbour's foot. We are continually aware of the presence of our fellow dancers. The group becomes a single entity and we are truly one. The steps are simple and small, with a meditative quality which allows us to immerse ourselves in the experience.

An Israeli dance introduces the concept of the group being a receptacle, a chalice, to receive and use the energy of the spirit. In the first part we each make a cup shape with our hands and there is a feeling of allowing it to be filled. It is slow and contemplative, an act of worship almost. Then there is a complete contrast as we run round the circle: for me this is the hustle and bustle of everyday life. Yet it is sustained and revitalised by the calm and precise nature of the receiving of spirit in the chalice. The teacher from whom I learnt this dance, used to describe it as "going to church and then going down the pub afterwards" and I am sure you will understand the meaning behind this comment. These are both group activities and they bring a balance into our lives: we may all have different ways of providing these contrasts, but we certainly do all need the counterpoise of rest and activity, of receiving and giving, of spirit and matter.

We believe that the most important aspect of a group of people working together is to acknowledge and celebrate the diversity of talent and ability represented by the members. We are all aiming at a common goal yet we will all bring different aptitudes to achieving that task. Each must be honoured for their very particular contribution. This lies behind good management and in my opinion is sadly lacking in the business world today. People seem to me to be treated as if they are all the same; there is little encouragement of individual expression, and frustration and lack of commitment to the goal are the inevitable result.

So, to celebrate and experience the diversity within the group we dance Menoussis from Greece. This has a basic sequence of steps which is the underlying theme. In my analogy it might be the overall goal. Within this there are a number of variations which the dancers are free to experience whenever they want to. We thus demonstrate our individuality within the common purpose — our diversity in unity. The person who chooses to continue with the basic step throughout is just as important in this dance as the one who is flamboyant and performs a variation every time. It is a question, in extreme expression, of valuing the tea-maker as much as the entrepreneur: each has their own unique talent which is necessary for the successful operation of the team. (As a little aside, Richard often says that counsellors were not necessary in the days of the tea lady! Everybody went to her with their problems and she just listened. The automatic drinks machine is not quite the same. So everybody has their talent and it may not be what they are outwardly in the group for.)

When we ran this workshop in Ireland someone made a very interesting comment: "Watching what others were doing threw me out; concentrating on my own interpretation, all was OK". Is this the essence of being in a group? We are aware of the presence of the other members, but if we spend too much time worrying about what they are doing, watching them, we lose our own purpose and enjoyment in the task.

So to the last dance in the spirit of the group, in which we explore group interaction and individuality in a slightly more ordered framework in the Dance of Unity. We move from one group to another and then find ourselves with space on our own. During that time we can do what we like — turn round on ourselves, hold our hands across our hearts, gently sway in time with the music — but, as I say, it is much like life — we only have four beats to do it in and then we are back into the next part of the dance. It does feel like that sometimes does it not? A moment of time to yourself soon vanishes as the next job has to be done, the next meeting attended.

This dance involves an interesting interweaving of two groups. We start off in two circles of equal size, one with hands joined moving synchronously and the other as individuals on the outside, free to express themselves however they wish. We then become one circle as the outside group links hands in front of the inside one. Thus we effortlessly combine forces: we are united as a bigger group. Finally those that were originally on the inside move outward and are on their own, while the second group moves to the centre and takes on the role of inner circle. The two sets interchange positions continuously joining forces in between the two extremes. It is yet another example of the cyclic nature of life.

In the discussion period on one occasion there was a recognition in the group that being a spiritual warrior can be lonely: being part of a group gives the individual support and shows how much fun it can be. "Feeling lonely is easier if you're not alone." There is an inner companionship which makes it very difficult to stay out on your own; but, as this dance illustrates, it would also be difficult for the group if anyone dropped out — in fact the dance would not work!

The music for this final dance is "Adoramus te Domine", a chant from the Taizé community in France where singing is a major part of worship. It is a group activity which enhances the sense of community spirit, and so it is used here in this workshop. It is a gentle, meditative and hypnotic piece which requires a period of quiet contemplation afterwards.

Meditation and discussion

We conclude with a meditation on the group as a circle of 'connectedness' in which each remains an individual and yet is drawn together for the common purpose of celebrating the spirit in a material world. We reflect on the idea of the group being a receptacle through which the divine may approach humanity and be directed out, inspiring others to service. In the "Affirmation of Group Unity"[20] we reinforce the strength of working together to a single purpose; the support that we can give to each other; and the power of the group to focus spiritual energy.

The discussion following this brief exploration of the spirit of the group often confirms the bond that has been created between members of the dancing circle. It emphasises for us the power of the dances to bring together disparate personalities in that sense of unity which honours and respects each individual and recognises the ability of the group to transcend human differences in a common purpose. This has always impressed me in Sacred Circle Dance and I believe that it can be an important tool in the future for generating this atmosphere in many settings where people meet together to undertake a single task.

---

20.   Copies of the "Affirmation of Group Unity" are available from World Goodwill, Suite 54, 3 Whitehall Court, London SW1A 2EF.

Human interaction

We have recognised the presence of divinity in and around us; we have
created a feeling of well-being and unity with our fellow dancers; we now
have to prepare for our journey back into everyday life. We have felt the
power of spirit within the group, we must now see how to retain it outside the confines of the hall and the workshop. Simply, we look at how to
live it.

The dances we use here are full of celebration: they are energetic.
After two or three dances in this part one participant said, "Gosh, it's
exhausting living it isn't it?"! Well, yes, maybe it is. Yet these lively dances
also *give* us energy to carry out our mission in life. They illustrate both
what is needed and what is available to us if we are to "live an ordinary
life in a non-ordinary way". Surely, if we are following the right path we
will be given that which we need to fulfil our role.

One dance emphasises the complexity of interacting with other people, the need to move from one to the next, giving and taking as we go.
We whirl round in pairs at one point and find that it is easier and we do
not become giddy if we look at each other. This is truly symbolic: if we
really interact with each other, look into each other's eyes and get to know
each other, the relationship becomes easier. We know the other person at
a deep level rather than merely as "ships that pass in the night".

Mori Shej is a delightful Hungarian gypsy dance: the song is to a
beloved baby daughter. I feel that here we experience paradox in dance!
The steps seem to be so simple (and they are) but it is extremely easy to
go wrong, particularly if you think about it too much. There are two sequences of steps both of which end with a 'side, tap' in each direction:
the confusion arises because the second part also starts with a 'side, tap'.
If we let our minds analyse it there seems to be a doubt as to whether to
do another side, tap: the feet are unsure where to go next, and confusion
reigns. Let go of the need to think about it and we sail along with the
music, being taken on a carefree journey of joy.

So too in life, if we analyse our actions and their consequences too
much we stumble and are unsure where we are heading. If we can let go
and trust the process of life it changes our attitude towards the 'problems'. We learn as we go. Is this the essence of a spiritual life? Maybe it is
about being prepared to make mistakes, even rejoicing in them because
thus we can develop. We are back to perfection not being perfect! We
have to keep a sense of proportion here: we cannot expect to do everything right the first time. The dances teach us that, if nothing else. We
have to keep practising; when we go wrong we learn something about
ourselves.

One participant, on losing the steps the second time through, asked himself in the context of the day: "Having experienced the Divine, how can we retain it?". Such a deep question from such a simple dance. Time and time again we witness the dances raising issues of this nature in people's minds: of course, we cannot answer all the questions — everyone has to find their own solution anyway — but we are confident that the dances will put a new perspective on life and generate stimulating discussion.

Goodwill

We also learn to co-operate with our fellow dancers. This is absolutely essential in my opinion in the greater aspect of the outside world. In the dance of life we necessarily come into contact with others who may not be hearing the same tune, or may have learnt different steps. We must attempt to adapt, to hear the other music, in order to understand each other and work together. Yet we must still listen to our rhythm and maintain our own integrity. It is a hard path to tread sometimes, but nevertheless rewarding.

In living a spiritual life in a material world we are called on to practice goodwill towards others, to exercise right human relations and indeed right relations with the whole of nature. In dance we experience this feeling of harmony with others, of enjoying each other's company. We make allowances for those that struggle with the steps. After all, we struggle ourselves too. If it is possible in a circle in which we know nobody, surely we can also create this atmosphere of goodwill in the diverse situations in which we find ourselves every day? We all have our difficulties: equally we can all help each other.

Perhaps I should define here what I mean by goodwill. I see it as the energy that makes right relations possible. It is a quality that is a prerequisite for peace in the world and in our communities. It is active. It has to be lived and made manifest. Goodwill can therefore be seen as the fundamental expression of spiritual living: "...goodwill is the touchstone that will transform the world."[21]

People often comment that it is easier to do a dance with the hands joined than to drop the handhold and move individually. There is safety in being a single unit, and there is mutual support. The energy flows round the circle and learning is facilitated. One beginner in a circle of experienced dancers may feel awkward at first but soon finds the benefit of their position: the circle will 'carry' the novice and the learning curve is

---

21.   Alice A Bailey, *Discipleship in the New Age*, vol I (Lucis Press Ltd, London) p. 65.

shortened. The goodwill of those who 'know' the dance towards the one who is new has been instrumental in making it a good experience. Again we can translate this into our 'normal' lives and help our fellow travellers along the way. We cannot learn the lessons for them but we can be of assistance by our attitude towards them.

Right human relations

The meditation at the end of this stage of the workshop is on this subject of goodwill. We reflect on our relationship with our family and friends, our community, our nation, the world of nations, the one humanity. We affirm this global connectedness. We visualise the energy of love flowing from the source of light, love and spiritual power through all people of goodwill and in to human hearts and minds everywhere. We meditate on ways in which we can spread goodwill and help create right human relations. We emphasise the need to be practical and start with our immediate sphere of influence.

Consolidation

We have run this workshop over two days, allowing us to incorporate a couple of additional dances in each section and a time at the end for reflection on the whole process and to repeat dances that have particular meaning for the participants. We find that revisiting the dances in the order and context in which we first introduced them enables the initial experience to be recaptured and further insight to emerge. There is always time for discussion as the theme has such relevance to everyone.

The final meditation provides a recapitulation of the day and an opportunity for people to consolidate their experiences and insight within their own hearts and minds. We then say together "The Great Invocation",[22] pausing between each stanza to reflect on the meaning of the words for us individually.

---

22. Copies of "the Great Invocation" are available from World Goodwill, Suite 54, 3 Whitehall Court, London SW1A 2EF

From the point of Light within the Mind of God
Let light stream forth into the minds of men.
Let Light descend on Earth.

From the point of Love within the Heart of God
Let love stream forth into the hearts of men.
May Christ return to Earth.

From the centre where the Will of God is known
Let purpose guide the little wills of men —
The purpose which the Masters know and serve.

From the centre which we call the race of men
Let the Plan of Love and Light work out
And may it seal the door where evil dwells.

Let Light and Love and Power restore the Plan on Earth.

I know there are some who find these words problematic because of the lack of mention of women. Indeed I have felt that way myself. I now believe that the beauty of the sentiments expressed goes way beyond our concern about gender. It is clear to me that the intention is to include the whole human race.

We conclude by sounding the Om three times. This is always an important moment for me: the room seems to vibrate as we all chant the same word at our own pitch. With the first exhalation we send out love and understanding; with the second, light; and with the third, power and the will-to-good. We are in unison and in harmony, truly celebrating the spirit in a material world.

Living it

The end of the day brings the greatest challenge as this is the time when we really have to go out and live it. Can we retain this feeling of goodwill and really make the changes we would like to see? Can we experience the 'unity in diversity' that the dances helped us to recognise? Can we always 'celebrate the spirit in a material world'?

The last dance is the same as the first: we conclude with "Song of the Soul": it is an uplifting dance that assists us in our endeavours. It leaves us in the centre in a position of aspiration, yet with a great shout of joy and accomplishment. At the end we feel, "Yes, all those things *are* possible".

Transition from the Old to the New

Richard

A fundamental aspect of the human experience is evolution. Nature, which we are part of, is constantly on the move, seeking new adaptations and passing through phases of metamorphosis. Thus life as we experience it is a continuum of transition, of change and of movement. The result is that the future becomes difficult to predict. It is not a clockwork universe: science reminds us that there is a fundamental uncertainty at the core of the building blocks of matter. Even at the macrocosmic level of human experience we find it difficult to predict future events with any great certainty. Always there are variables that cannot be pinned down and which ensure the unexpected is always just around the next corner!

Transition requires movement. In so far as transition in time is concerned, this may well mean making choices as to what to leave behind in the past, and what to embrace in the future. This might involve jobs, relationships, hobbies. It could mean changes in mind-set and philosophical viewpoint. It will probably involve loss *and* gain. It will certainly involve choice.

We found ourselves in 1995 wondering whether to run another alternative Christmas Day, or perhaps explore the meaning of New Year. We had both been pondering on the nature of transition and why it is such a crucial factor in the human experience, yet one that is not always focused on as an issue in its own right. It seemed so obvious that New Year was the time to explore this topic. The workshop began to take shape in our minds and took form as 'Transition from the Old to the New' on 31 December 1995.

Yet transition is ever present; so its implications can be explored at any time of year. If you think about it, at whatever point we are in life we are experiencing transition, because no part of our present is permanent. We are always moving from one place to another, whether externally or internally.

For some people the current transition that is of major significance may be to do with relationships, or perhaps their job. It could be that something from the past is to be let go of, or there is a need to adjust to accommodate a fresh vision of the future they seek to create. We might see our lives as a continuum of transitions, some taking years, others occurring in an instant. Indeed, breathing is an ever-present transition, as we breathe in and then breathe out. The blood coursing through the arteries and veins expresses a cyclic transition as the heart expands and contracts to pump it round.

Many transitions do not seem to unsettle us, they have been accepted as normal — day/night, the seasons of the year. They have a degree of certainty. We know where we are with them, although the pattern of weather seems to be more uncertain these days in many people's minds.

Transition is a theme that is with us every moment of the day, even though we generally try to avoid thinking about it. Indeed, all is constantly moving and changing and each moment truly is the only reality we ever have. Yet how much time is spent dwelling on the past: either out of guilt or shame about something we feel we should not have done, or with a smile as we remember good times and lose ourselves in reminiscence. Or anticipating the future: either fearfully as to what might happen, or with anticipation and expectation of what tomorrow may hold for us. Whilst the poor old present, the only moment we ever really have, gets forgotten or ignored (Figure 25). The present becomes lost to the past, to be replaced by another present, which if we are not careful will suffer the same fate as the last one.

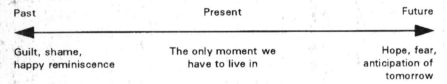

Past	Present	Future
Guilt, shame, happy reminiscence	The only moment we have to live in	Hope, fear, anticipation of tomorrow

Figure 25. The struggle to keep your eye on the present

What we seek to achieve during the workshop is to provide a space for people to explore and experience transition and to watch themselves sharing in activities that involve movement from one action to the next in a variety of contexts. Sometimes it may be that we are driven to change, at other times we are more measured and in control. Sometimes there is a sense of direction and yet at other times it is blind.

Life is rather like going on a journey. Some of us, though, are so one-pointed towards arriving at the destination that we forget to look out of the window and experience the journey itself. Traffic jams can be awfully irritating, but once you accept you are stuck and it really does not matter what you do you are not going to get to that meeting, you can sit back, turn off the mobile phone and enjoy the opportunity for some space of your own. It does not have to be a stressful experience if you let go of your fretting about the future and where you should be, and simply accept where you are, stuck in a transition jam! Time to slot in that new language tape, or the recorded book you never got round to reading. Find time for yourself.

Global transition

We begin the workshop with a dance that itself is full of transition, in which the group moves through a variety of handholds, opening up and closing down, giving us space to expand and to stretch and then to move back into a much tighter and containing relationship.

We spend the first session of the day considering transition on a global scale. We use dances from diverse cultures to illustrate change and movement. The first is about being stuck in the indecision of transition, enabling us to rush to and fro, using lots of energy and enthusiasm, but not actually getting anywhere! Does this sound like life? We also use a dance that is concerned with community building after war. It is a women's dance from Greece and powerfully takes us on a journey of mutual support to a turning outwards back into the world. Part of the dance requires us to hold hands facing the centre, then we turn to face out, bringing a very different feel. Are we secure enough to face out into the world? The dance alternates between looking inwards and outwards, providing a powerful experience of transition and contrast.

From here we move to a community-building dance from Israel — a troubled part of the world in which races of people struggle to establish their own community and cultural identity, and yet ancient divisiveness obstructs the expansion of this identity to embrace a multi-cultural reality. The music for this dance was recorded by us in Tel Aviv with our friend playing her accordion.

Early in 1996, after the bus bombing in Tel Aviv, I called our friends to see if they were alright. Re-experiencing this dance, which we learned and recorded in their small living room in down-town Tel Aviv, brought back the memory of that phone-call and hearing the sounds of the sirens of the emergency vehicles in the background. It has left me knowing that personal contact with people from other countries and cultures is incredibly important. It can hurt to know and love people in troubled areas of the world, but it certainly stops you from ever feeling compassion fatigue. If we all knew someone personally from every country we could be taking a big step towards a better and more humane future.

Our final dance, from India, highlights the role of the creator and the destroyer as represented by Shiva, and the drawing in and breathing out of the spirit by the disciple on the journey towards enlightenment. Transition is about death and rebirth, about moving on. It is also concerned with sacrifice, maybe a particular activity or a way of thinking, or an habitual reaction to a situation. Yet sacrifice is more than destroying a form. The word sacrifice is from the root *sacer*, meaning sacred, and *facere*, to make. When we sacrifice something in the sense of giving it up, are we not also releasing ourselves and the object of our sacrifice in order to move on? In this light we might view transition as an opportunity to move towards greater holiness or wholeness. In transition we give *of* ourselves in order to bridge the past and future. We experience the moment to the extent that we give of ourselves in the moment. We are the bridge all the time. In this way we live the life of the disciple.

The aim of the morning is to bring us to a sense of the challenge of transition and to become sensitive to the 'flow of experiencing' that passes through us. We then use this sensitivity to focus on the global situation, as affairs on planet Earth are certainly in a state of flux and transition. Participants value this. By placing our own sense of transition within that greater context we can generate fresh perspectives, ideas and motivation to contribute to change for the better.

Everywhere there is change and adjustment. There are forces seeking to cling to old ways, others seeking the new at the expense of the traditional. People with extreme views exist in all areas of life as do those holding positions at every point between them.

As we view world problems, many argue that a little positive thought and meditation on its own can change things. Well, energy does follow thought as far as I am concerned, and I do feel that we are witnessing what amounts to a global meditation as leading thinkers and people of goodwill strive to formulate intelligent solutions to world problems. We try to emphasise the need for practical action to flow from our reflective thinking. We need to consider in our hearts and minds what we can usefully, collectively leave behind as we move away from the past: attitudes rooted in a separative identity, greed, selfishness and a willingness to exploit; the insular and nationalistic pattern of political and economic life; the refusal to show tolerance towards people of different beliefs.

It is important for us to know what we aspire to leave behind, but we must also put our thought to what we will take with us as the basis for creation in the future. What principles do we wish to see the human community adopt? Sharing? Selflessness? Tolerance? Environmental sensitivity? We must also then ask what must we do in the present to enable these attitudes to become the bedrock of a future reality. Hence the need to be practical, to consider what we can each do within our own areas of interest, service and responsibility to carry the vision of a better way into everyday life.

It is often said that we cannot change the world until we change ourselves. There is a certain truth in this, but there is a demon in it too. If we wait for personal change to happen we may never engage in the challenge of world service. Wherever we live we are all surrounded by human need and there is no excuse for not doing anything to help lift the human condition. Waiting to be inspired before we serve is to put the coach before the horse. We grow by experience, and the experience of service, of courageously playing our part in the human drama, brings us the really great lessons of life.

Personal change

During the afternoon session we concentrate more on personal change and growth. We explore transition in time, how we often lose sight of the present moment because we are dwelling on the past or expectant of the future. We use a dance that takes us back and forth as if we are looking to the past and into the future and at the end of each sequence we find we have moved around the circle. Yet we have very little sense of having made that movement.

An interesting discussion arose on one occasion about the nature of change — is it a process or an event? It seems to depend on the length of time during which the change takes place. Either way it can be difficult. We find ourselves struggling to adjust fast enough when the event is sudden, yet when we experience a slow process of transition we can be uncomfortable with the on-going period of change and uncertainty.

We use one dance that is in reality a combination of two, with a sudden change in the middle, and then a return to the first dance. Even though we know it is coming, the transition seems still to take us unawares and a period of chaos ensues as we try to let go of the old rhythm and adjust to the new. Then, just as we get the hang of that, the dance goes back to its original form! Some people spend the whole dance anticipating the change and therefore not fully experiencing the present moment. Others can be free of this and simply worry about the adjustment when the change occurs. Our experience of the dance can be an indicator of how we approach change in life. Do we constantly worry about it, allowing our anticipation to affect our present, or can we feel secure enough in ourselves to know we can live the present to the full and adjust when necessary?

We also dance into stages of life, comparing an old woman moving slowly and reflectively with her style of dance when she was young. You may recognise this description from the earlier chapter on 'Beyond Balance — Towards Complementarity'. Yes, we sometimes use the same dances in different contexts. In 'Beyond Balance' this dance serves to contrast the 'opposites' of old and young: in this workshop, however, our focus is on the experience of transition that arises as we move from one state to another. How quickly can we adapt to changes of speed? How does it feel in that moment of transition?

It is fascinating how using the same dance but with a shift in emphasis can change the experience of the movements and the feelings it generates. This applies to even the simplest of dances: someone who has been attending Lynn's evening classes regularly for many years and now leads her own groups, came to one of our workshops for the first time. She was amazed how much more she began to see in the dances that were really familiar to her: it altered her concept of Sacred Circle Dance and its power.

This comes out well in a Hungarian gypsy dance we use to experience the confusion of transition. Again this is a dance we have used in another workshop to capture the celebratory nature of living spiritually. It is a simple, rhythmic dance yet it seems forever to go back and forward in a rhythm that at times we flow with and then we somehow get one step wrong and we are heading off in the wrong direction! However, whereas earlier dances seemed to dominate us and drive us along, here there is scope for imposing ourselves on the dance to bring our own style into the movement. Sometimes we are pushed into and through transition, like a swimmer caught by strong waves and currents; at other times we have just enough distance from the forces at work in our lives to ride the transition, rather like a surfer on a wave, maintaining his or her balance on the surfboard. A very different experience.

Running this event over New Year fits well with all the talk about New Year resolutions. Indeed, it provides an opportunity maybe to share these with others and to gain strength and inspiration as a result. In the middle of the afternoon we offer a ritual in which we write the qualities, experiences or facets of our lives that we wish to leave behind, and those that we wish to see present in the future. We set fire to the old, burning it away, ritualistically releasing ourselves. Some people also like to burn the new. This is their choice.

It is worth considering what contributes to successful resolutions, and why it is that so many fail. Failure is very often linked to resolutions being either totally unrealistic or simply unplanned. We have to plan change in order to give it a chance of becoming established. Habits of a lifetime do not just vanish into thin air. We have to think through what we hope to achieve, gain a sense of what threatens our process of change, and seek ways of reducing these threats. We also need to plan new elements in our life to replace what we are seeking to leave behind. Should you find your resolution does not hold, do not just give up in the belief that you do not have the will power: explore it and give yourself the chance to understand why it did not work out. Maybe something can be learned that will make the next attempt successful.

Cycle of change

I generally spend a little time at this stage of the workshop talking about my work as an alcohol counsellor and how we help and support people in making change happen. I believe this can be usefully applied to New Year resolutions and, indeed, to anything that we feel we want to change in our lives. The model I talk about is a version of one formulated in the 1980s specifically for people with addictive problems (Figure 26).

According to this model, when we are involved in making changes in our lives, we pass through a series of stages. We may be at a point of not wanting to change our habitual pattern in some area of our life. However, something may happen to cause us to question this, and we move to a stage of thinking about change. During this phase, we will probably weigh up the pros and cons. Having decided to alter an established habit, we then begin to plan how we can bring this about. The next stage is to put this plan into action, followed by a period of seeking to maintain the change. It may become established and we will exit the cycle of change having achieved our goal. On the other hand, we may relapse: as a result we may give up and exit the cycle of change completely, or we may explore why relapse occurred and begin to formulate a new action plan.

I believe that many New Year resolutions 'fail' because they have been unplanned and there is no appreciation that we learn from relapse, that it does not have to be a time of giving up, but of trying again — this time a little wiser.

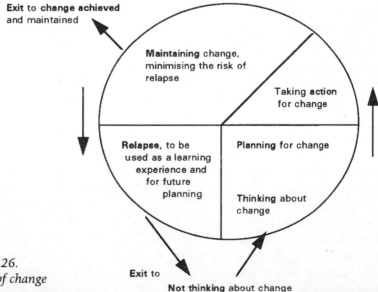

Figure 26.
Cycle of change

When we achieve our goal we may feel so empowered by the experience that we begin to question other areas of our life. We may then begin to formulate new action plans to bring about further changes.

It reminds me how, some years back, I struggled to walk past the confectionery kiosk at Embankment station in London each morning on my way to work without going and buying a chocolate bar. It may sound a little thing but I experienced some of the symptoms of addiction as I tried to avoid temptation: the little voice goading me into 'just the one', and, 'you can stop tomorrow'; anxiety and a real sense of loss and discomfort. I guess part of it had been a reward for the journey and I wanted my reward. Yet it can be overcome by will-power, but there are other ways: getting off at a different station, taking a different route so you do not pass the places that you associate with the habit. A little bit of strategic planning can make a lot of difference! Of course, I did not know all this then and I rather feel that I probably just transferred my need for a comforting chocolate bar to a need for a comforting doughnut later in the day!

Embracing the new

To return to the workshop, after our ritual burning away of the old and welcoming in the new, we enter the final stage — celebrating the new. We use dances that involve change but also have a celebratory energy to them. The first, from Russia, conveys a sense of changing direction with confidence and purpose, joy and steadiness. Then we enter a quite different experience through an African dance that is truly a celebration of life in which we move individually with a lot of bodily expression, arm waving and clapping! Great fun!

We then move on to a dance in which we can choose our own steps during some sections. Perhaps our journey of transition has been about learning to make choices for ourselves, or to be a little more individual and expressive. This dance offers an opportunity to test this out, in a safe environment. Finally we share in a dance that encompasses a recognition of the past, the joy and exhilaration of throwing ourselves into the experience of the now, and a willingness to move on enthusiastically to new experiences.

The aim of this section is really to get people into a celebratory experience and to engage with the energy of the new. People describe an increase in motivation and a greater zest for life.

We share in a short visualisation based around an affirmation that I wrote some years back, which I believe carries power and direction and serves to offer each participant an opportunity to engage with their own sense of direction.

The Way Ahead

I am the Soul.
There is no Self apart to do my work for me,
No splendid being to take my rebellious nature in hand.
I must control my outer form and life and all events.
I, the Soul, the true Self, am
And no-one can take that reality from me.

Look to yourself.
Take heart, take courage and take control.
Drive on into the cold clear light.
Burn into being.
Naught can hinder the one who treads the path of fire.

Forward and upward. Inward and outward.
All ways are one Way.
The path behind is no longer yours to tread.
Leave it for those who follow on.

Prepare the way.
Stand,
Yet onward move.
You are. All is. Move on.

Finally, we repeat the opening dance but this time, rather than ending it in a tight circle and a front basket-weave handhold, we end standing further apart with our hands raised above us. Now, commanding our own space, we can take that next step of returning with renewed energy and purpose to engage with life.

Living with uncertainty

One of the things that concerns us about transition is that it reminds us that life is uncertain and that with all the best planning and insurance the world can give us, there is always the probability of the unexpected happening. Indeed, the more secure we try to make our lives, maybe the more likely that we will experience the unexpected. Well, we have not got room for anything else when everything is so planned and structured! It is also worth noting how if we were to try to plan our lives right down to the merest detail in order to try to remove, or cater for, uncertainty, we would actually be creating a very false sense of security. The unexpected can still happen, and if it does against a background of so much careful planning then it is going to be an even greater shock!

Some people spend their time seeking to create a secure way of living. They do not know the essence of human life that is rooted in uncertainty. They seek to generate an environment that brings them comfort and security. They seek to know 'where they stand' in all matters that arise. They seek to be sure, to be in a position to maintain control over their destinies and their environments. They seek order — their order — in all that they experience. They tread a path that is contrary to the nature of Reality, a path that in truth is one of foolishness.

Others accept, indeed embrace, uncertainty. They know that they cannot create a lasting security which can be imposed upon their lives or anyone else's. They realise that each moment is a fresh creative opportunity rich with infinite possibilities which calls them to fulfil the duty of the hour. They know that outer order is a temporary condition. It will pass. The knowledgeable do not cling to the passing order, their concern is not with the temporal. They live to the truth of uncertainty, the reality of life on Earth.

For humanity, the great illusion of our time is the search for order, security and certainty in all things. This illusion will pass. It may be that it manifests through a desire to restore the perceived order of the past. It may be through the desire to establish a new order for the future. Either way, it is rooted in desire. Order born out of desire has no reality in truth and it will always manifest with its accompanying opposite — disorder. All action out of desire manifests in a duality of experience.

Why do we put so much creative energy into establishing order? Because it is more comfortable — and less risky (or so we think). Let us, though, put aside our desires for order, either from the past or for the future. Let us rise above it and realise that the only secure future is rooted in embracing Life, and where Life interacts with humanity it manifests as uncertainty. If we are to Know Life we must accept uncertainty, and embrace the not-knowing of living.

The paradox is (and in life there is always a paradox), when we do accept uncertainty, when we dance to the unknown rhythm, we discover order. It is a higher order, an order not of our making. It is an order that is willed-to-be by a much greater Creative Life. Such an order will come for us all. It will be known by more and more people, and by you and me.

When, of course, is uncertain. Perhaps today, perhaps tomorrow, perhaps in a hundred years' time, but it will come. Not through the workings of our desire to impose some partial human order upon our world, but through our ability to accept and live with uncertainty. By embracing uncertainty we allow that Greater Life to live through us in each creative moment.

Living with uncertainty does not mean we do not plan ahead. Rather, our planning is flexible and open to embracing fresh opportunities. Now, this can be taken to the extreme of leaving your options so open that you do nothing. So often this approach to life does not work, simply because it is rooted in fear: fear of missing out on something, usually, or of making the 'wrong' choice. In such things there is no right and wrong, merely the treading of a path through life that will bring us experience and opportunities to share who and what we are with others. We cannot keep every option open, we have to make choices. The trick lies in not getting too attached to the form of life, in accepting the transience of form, and in placing our emphasis on the quality of our life.

The great transition many would say is death. If we know the impermanence of form, and the immortality of the Soul, what is there to fear? We sleep and awaken in another room. Life goes on though the form may change. We each have our own beliefs which we generate as we travel through life to help us make sense of our experiences. For me, only one crack at life seems futile. What would be the point? Is life only about the evolution of forms through natural selection and survival of the fittest? Is my body and what it passes on to the next generation all that is important about my years on Earth? To me, that does not make sense, it does not add up. The idea of progressive learning and an evolution of conscious being through a succession of forms to me makes sense. I guess I just have an in-built sense of continuity.

From the old to the new

It is really worthwhile stopping for a moment and considering what we carry with us from the past. Maybe we have learned to see ourselves, or others, in a particular light that obscures our ability to see clearly in the present? Perhaps we avoid certain situations or experiences because of a bad time we had in similar circumstances many years ago. Or we may readily embrace relationships that for us are normal, but only because we have never had the opportunity to experience anything different and therefore make an informed choice.

Even in seemingly insignificant things we can find ourselves loaded up with the past. Think of school dinners. I am sure that there is something that you really did not like but perhaps were forced to eat, and which you vowed never to go near again!

Working with transition is about being able to be free to make choices that are informed and truly independent of past associations. It is to do with bringing an air of liberation into what we undertake in the present. It is also about having a sense of direction and a willingness to create our own vision for the future. We may not get to it, we may end up taking another path, but we need vision and a goal to work towards. When we cannot look ahead we are in a desperate situation.

Imagine a visit from your fairy godmother: you have one wish, and it is to be made for something new to be part of your life that you know will fill you with anticipation and expectation; something that will make you want to get up and know it will be a good day because that which you have wished for is part of your life that day. Be realistic. Now, write it down. Next, ask yourself what you are already doing about making this treasured something part of your life. Finally, if you are not doing anything about it already, ask yourself "why not?". If it is something that important to you and it will really make a positive and fulfilling difference to your life, what is hindering you from already working towards it?

We need to begin to think this way if we are to work with transition and to participate in creating our own future rather than simply allowing ourselves to be pushed around by old habits and limited expectations. Life may be uncertain, and we may not be able to guarantee anything, but let us at least give ourselves a chance, an opportunity, to make choices, and to participate in bringing about the new that we would like to see as part of our personal life, family life, or maybe the life of the wider human family.

From the Love of Power to the Power of Love

Lynn

It was one of those 'chance' remarks — yet does anything really happen by chance? I am inclined to think not. I like the expression 'synchronistic'. I believe that whatever befalls is part of a plan that we are largely unaware of: things that appear to be 'coincidence' are in fact 'coincidence', or happening at the same time and at the same place. Our everyday language has corrupted the meaning of the word and therefore our expectation: 'coincidence' has come to mean 'purely by chance'. In my experience synchronicity is very much a part of life and the more we recognise it occurring, the more it will occur. It is as if a change in our mind-set, our acknowledgement of the magic in life, changes the reality.

We were nearing the end of a wonderful weekend in Cork investigating the Cross and the Circle: it was March and the sun had shone from the beginning to the end. We were in a South-facing room and had to have the windows open! Our hosts were bowled over by the weather, particularly as this had happened to us the year before as well. Then we had spent a whole week on the West coast in glorious sunshine: we had seen the tops of mountains that the locals declared could only be seen once in five years! Our view of Ireland is of a beautiful country bathed in sun, with incredible blue skies ... we have been very lucky.

So back to the last ten minutes of a weekend full of warmth, both outside and inside, stimulating discussions, and inspiring dancing. I cannot remember now what the remark was, but I do recall the certain knowledge that here was our next theme for a workshop. I looked across the circle at Richard, he nodded. We knew we had been given our next challenge. Ten minutes later I had the title — From the Love of Power to the Power of Love — it came to me in a flash and I could hardly wait to tell Richard.

An hour later we were driving from Cork to Rosslare to catch the ferry and we were already planning next year's visit to Ireland. Well, since that group had been the inspiration for the subject matter, they had to be the first to experience the outcome!

It has proved to be one of our most popular topics: the title from that moment of connection and conscious recognition has captured the imagination of many groups. As an example, we were invited to run this workshop in Dundee in May 1996. Afterwards we were asked to return in 1997 with another subject. When we were preparing our brochure for the first half of the year, we realised that, although we were fairly sure which theme had been chosen, we had not actually written it down. When we rang the organiser, he had had the same problem when preparing his programme. He was running out of time and made a quick decision without asking us: he felt the title 'From the Love of Power to the Power of Love' said so much that he chose to run that one again!

Once more we found the content of the workshop falling quite naturally into that magic number three. First we investigate the many faces of power, then different aspects of love, and finally we bring the two together and look at how love can be used as a force for good in the world.

We consider it to be a journey through the stage of love of self and the discovery of personal power, to the realisation of a greater love whose power knows no bounds. The world needs strong, powerful people with a loving and compassionate vision: in dance we can experience these qualities and know how it feels to possess them.

Faces of power and love

We start with a 'brainstorm' of the many faces of power and love. It is interesting to find that some qualities come up in both: strength, for instance, is considered an aspect of power and also part of love. It is fascinating to see different words coming out in the various groups: they seem to reflect the feelings within the participants. Often the power words are fairly negative, even representing an element of fear: words such as dominating, inhibiting and authority are common. On the other hand love seems to conjure up good feelings with words such as gentleness, caring and healing.

There seems to be an idea abroad that power is bad and love is good. Many people these days try to deny the power side of their character and focus solely on love. While this may lead to a world in which love is paramount, I believe it is also very unbalanced. With only love, there is no impulse to do anything: it is power or will that drives us to express love. It is an essential element of our lives; we deny it at our peril. In the workshop we often have to remind people to consider the positive aspects of power as well as the frightening and domineering ones. Equally we may steer the group away from the rather 'wishy-washy' qualities of love towards those stronger, more determined aspects.

It is an interesting process to watch: the realisation that our preconceived ideas about two small words in our language can lead us to a very biased view of life. Then the acknowledgement that there are two sides to both words: one is certainly not all bad, neither is the other all good. It is no better to smother someone in love than it is to act in a totalitarian way towards others.

Aspects of power

The flipchart pages soon fill up and we leave them out for people to consider or to augment during the workshop. We move on to dancing some of the many aspects of personal power. We begin with a dance that comes from the time of the colonels in Greece: the title means, "What more is there to say?" It is a very simple dance which gives a real sense of standing up for ourselves against all adversity. The movements are deliberate, purposeful and we are left with a feeling of growing a couple of inches. We stand more upright at the end. We are strong.

Something that fascinates me about this dance is that the phrasing of the steps is not the same as that of the music: this is not uncommon in Greek dances but it is particularly poignant because of the meaning we are attaching to it. We move 'against' the music, occasionally the steps start at the beginning of a phrase in the tune, but more often they are totally out of 'synch'. In our interpretation for this workshop we talk of the need sometimes to maintain our own power even when we are moving out of kilter with others. We have to stand firm with our own beliefs and in the end the music and the dance finish at the same time! We can learn so much from this kind of simple experience.

Next we look at the idea of 'power over' others. This is a difficult concept for some: it is not a quality that we necessarily want to cultivate. It is something most people are very frightened of both in themselves and in others, yet we have to acknowledge that it is a part of our lives. There is a Greek brigands' dance that demonstrates this very well. I believe that it is much better to experience these types of feelings in dance than in the outside world. If we dance this face of power, we know the buzz it might give, but nobody suffers as a result.

The brigands are moving round their captives and at one point become quite threatening. A menacing sequence towards the centre, followed by a shout and a kicking retreat would leave the victims terrified. I once taught this dance from the centre of the circle and had to beat a very hasty retreat as my 'captors' proceeded viciously towards me! Usually it is a wonderful experience to be in the centre of the circle but not in this dance. Yet, when we were in Poland in 1996, some people wanted to find out what it felt like in the middle. I tried to dissuade them but they were adamant. We danced round them; we approached the centre with our best brigand visage; and we kicked our way back out again. At the end of the dance they were totally unmoved! I think the group was so cohesive by that time in the week that our 'captives' could not feel any threat from their 'captors'. I still would not recommend sitting in the centre for this one though.

Another wonderful experience we had with this dance was again in Poland with a different group of people. One man found it particularly empowering. There was no way he wanted to go out and exert power over other people but he found a means of giving himself strength to balance his own gentleness and artistic nature. It was a real revelation to us to see this happening before our very eyes.

Our third dance is very different: it is a gentle floating dance. How does this fit into the concept of power? The first time we ran this workshop someone said: "I thought you would use that dance but I expected it to be for love". Yes power and love are closely connected. Richard and I had debated long about it: we moved this dance from the power of love section to love and finally put it in power. What clinched it was that it is done without joining hands. We dance as individuals and can each move how we want to within the restriction of the basic steps and the confines of the circle. We are encouraged to move gracefully with power within our own space.

There are four sequences of three beats. The first two movements have a certain hesitation and preparation about them. In the third set of steps we cross our hands in front and then in the fourth bar we turn round on ourselves leading with the right arm. It is a wonderful moment of liberation, a letting go of pent-up energy and a feeling of strength despite the apparent gentleness of the movement.

On one occasion my next door neighbour in this dance said afterwards that at first he felt intimidated by my energy in doing this final movement. He then realised that it was up to him to take control of the situation for himself and he claimed his own space and began to enjoy the dance again. We both learned a lesson from those few moments and the honest sharing afterwards: I learned how easy it is unintentionally to invade someone else's space; my neighbour learned that he had control over his own reactions and actions. All this from one dance!

So we move on to animal power in another Greek dance in celebration of the bull. It is a wonderful piece of music with a very strong beat. In the dance we represent the horns of the bull, the front and back legs and the tail. We paw the ground, we flick the tail and can really feel the energy of the bull breathing 'fire'. To represent the animal's legs we jump to face the centre with the feet about shoulder width apart, knees bent, hands coming up quite sharply and purposefully with the biceps muscles tensed: it is certainly a powerful moment, which is followed by pawing the ground! Here is the raw animal power, unharnessed, waiting to be unleashed.

Another anecdote from Poland will illustrate how this can be tamed and used to our advantage. A friend in Warsaw had danced these power dances with us at both the summer camps in 1996. Soon afterwards she heard that she had to leave her flat right in the centre of Warsaw. She wanted to buy a place of her own (not at all easy in Poland — there is still not much privately owned property and there is not the same concept of mortgages). We spoke to her on the phone and she told us that she was using the power dances, and in particular the bull dance, to gain her own personal power for the difficult period ahead of her, which would include discussing money and loans with financial wizards — not something which she was used to or enthusiastic about! What a very positive and affirming way to use these dances: this is dance in action, creating an atmosphere in which difficulties can be overcome and we can take our own power again.

Finally we do a Macedonian dance which becomes fast and sometimes a little chaotic. It is persistent; the energy builds up and we move diagonally into the centre and out again; we feel the air rush past us as we go in; nothing can stop us; nothing gets in our way. Gradually the speed builds up, the intensity of the music increases and we end up totally exhilarated and exhausted all at the same time. How like the buzz some people have when they are in the position of power. They drive themselves and everybody else (for in this dance we are most certainly joined and what one does the others do too) almost to the point of collapse. In business, relentless drive may lead a person to having an ulcer or a heart attack, or giving one to their colleagues. The buzz and the burn out are both important aspects of power. Sometimes we need this form of power to *break through* and achieve some demanding task, yet it can put us at risk of *breakdown*.

Sharing

Time now for sharing feelings about the dances. We also have a number of quotations which we have found about power. At this stage it is sometimes necessary to bring in a lighter note so we may concentrate on some less serious aspects of power — or are they? Shaw in his inimitable way has had some wonderful things to say about both power and love. For instance, from *The Man of Destiny*: "There is nothing so bad or so good that you will not find an Englishman doing it; but you will never find an Englishman in the wrong. He does everything on principle. He fights you on patriotic principles; he robs you on business principles; he enslaves you on imperial principles." One of my favourites is from Spock in *Star Trek*: "I object to intellect without discipline. I object to power without constructive purpose". Many a true word is spoken in the unlikeliest setting!

To end the session on power Richard leads a visualisation. We have based this on the Buddhist disidentification exercise with which you may be familiar. It starts "I have a body but I am not my body". The essence of it is to affirm our power over form: we each acknowledge that we have a body, emotions and a mind but that is not 'me'. Right at the end we affirm:

I am a centre of will and from this centre of true identity I can learn to observe, direct and harmonise all my psychological processes and my physical body. I will to achieve a constant awareness of this fact in the midst of my everyday life, and to use it to help me and give increasing meaning and direction to my life.

This seems to give a new meaning to personal power: it is no longer detrimental to others; it is a way by which we become complete human beings and can enrich our spiritual life.

Aspects of love

There are so many different aspects to love, yet we only have one word in the English language. It was difficult to make the decision as to which half dozen qualities we would choose to dance. We start with a woman's dance which emphasises the physical aspect of love, self-love, showing off to others. The music is lively and in the second part we go into the centre leading with the hips in a rather saucy, provocative movement. As the dance progresses the music speeds up and becomes quite exciting.

I have a wonderful picture in my mind as I write, of a male participant at one of our workshops who really got into this dance. His face was alight and he was thoroughly enjoying himself using his body in this unusual way. Those who truly enter into this dance find themselves quite exhausted at the end: it is tiring continually to present this lively, full-of-oneself attitude and we experience this directly in the dance.

Our second face of love is very different. It is that floaty, indefinable, transient love — the holiday romance that has that element of unreality about it. The dance we use is one that I choreographed many years ago for a very different purpose to Gheorge Zamfir's version of "Eté d'Amour" — a haunting tune on pan pipes that is reminiscent of sun-drenched days on sandy beaches with seagulls crying overhead.

The steps are simple, representing the uncomplicated nature of this type of relationship (until the holiday ends of course!). In fact there is basically only one sequence, with an interlude in the middle in which everybody has eight beats to move in and out of the centre however they want: this is done in two parts so that we make a choice as to whether to be in the first group or the second. There are three points in the dance when we are stationary, bending our knees in rhythm with the music, while lifting our hands up and then bringing them down. There is a feeling of flying away with the seagulls, of floating on the breeze. Indeed, we end with our hands in the air as if permanently transported.

We move on to a progressive partner dance from Russia, which gives us an experience of the goodwill aspect of love. We move together as one big circle, then split into pairs to greet each other, the left-hand partner walking round to the other side, making eye contact all the time. This introduces the idea of a love that is non-judgmental: we greet all our partners in the same way, concentrating on that one person out of all the group during those eight beats and then moving on to the next. It is a beautiful, simple representation of goodwill to all.

I am reminded of a quotation I heard recently which has left a lasting mark, yet I cannot remember who said it: "Strangers are friends we haven't met yet". So simple, so brief and so thought-provoking: our Russian partner dance captures this same sentiment.

The gentle, affectionate love of an uncle for his niece is represented in a slow Israeli dance which ends with a sequence in which we bend down to the earth as if picking up something: we then open our arms high above us as if offering that same something to a greater cause. It is the selfless love of a parent or, in the case of this particular song, an uncle for a child. It is the love that is prepared to make sacrifices for the other or on behalf of the other. Again the steps are simple although there are three patterns to master: the first sequence is repeated after each of the others as if bringing us back again each time to the basics of this uncomplicated love.

Sadly we have had two occasions on which this love has been misinterpreted. We hear so much today of child abuse and it seems that the love of an older man towards a young girl can be easily misconstrued. This is not, however, the meaning of the song, the dance or our use of it in this context. It is just what I have described: the love of an uncle for his niece.

Finally, another Israeli dance which is a real celebration of life and love. The title means "I have not yet loved enough" and the dance feels as if there is some urgency in remedying this! It is fast and exciting: we move to the left and then pause to give and receive by moving our hands, palms upwards, towards the centre, palms down as we retract them. Giving and receiving — so much a part of a real loving relationship. The second part of the dance sees us moving to the centre raising our hands high above us and then out again as our hands come back down, as if we are reaching up and bringing blessings down to earth. We then scatter them abroad in a final complete turn round ourselves. This is the love that gives us energy, that spurs us on to do more, to demonstrate our compassion and concern for others.

Effect of dances

When we sit down to talk about the effect the dances have had on us, it is surprising how often people talk of having experienced qualities that we would normally associate more with power: they feel good about themselves; they feel the strength in the self-sacrificing love; and the solidarity of greeting each other in the goodwill dance. This just shows us the power of love which we investigate next.

We have found some wonderful quotations about love. Again many of them are from Shaw. "It's not easy being in love with me is it? But it's good for you" (*Major Barbara*). There is one that we use just before lunch: "There is no love sincerer than the love of food" (*Man and Superman*). We find it important to intersperse the day with some humour: life can be very serious and laughing is a wonderful release.

We end this journey into love with a visualisation in which we each focus on a particular heart quality and imagine how we might apply it in our own lives. We then say a short affirmation which expresses powerful sentiments of love:

> In the centre of all love I stand
> From that centre I, the Soul, will outward move
> From that centre I, the one who serves, will work.
> May the love of the Divine Self be shed abroad
> In my heart, through my group, and throughout the world.[23]

We conclude by sounding the Om three times: the reverberation round the hall is beautiful; it feels to me as though I am in a world where there is only the Om — it vibrates within me around me and through me.

Aspects of the power of love

> The core of [Mani's] teaching was the conception that humanity was created in order to transform the evil in the universe through the power of love.

This is a quotation from *The Cup of Destiny* by Trevor Ravenscroft[24] when he is talking about Manichaean Christianity. This is an awesome responsibility yet we have already found in doing the love dances that they

---

23.   Copies of the "Affirmation of Love" are available from World Goodwill, Suite 54, 3 Whitehall Court, London SW1A 2EF.

24.   Trevor Ravenscroft, *The Cup of Destiny: the Quest for the Grail* (Rider & Co, London, 1981) p. 39.

generate a certain element of power. Love is a power, a source of strength and a vital force for good in the world.

In the Arthurian legends we hear a great deal about love and power. The sword itself was symbolic of both. In *The Symbolic Meaning of the Story of King Arthur* we read:

> The sword as a whole signified Power. The handle and pommel together were symbolical of Humility, and as these were the parts by which the weapon was controlled, Arthur was reminded that Power must always be used with Humility.[25]

In our case, perhaps, we can legitimately translate humility from this passage into love. So power on its own can be destructive. Love on its own can be selfish and introverted. Bring the two together and we can change the world for good.

In the stories of Arthur we see the knights proving their prowess with a lance: they charge forward without concern for their opponent (in many cases we read of battles in which the two contestants did not know who they were fighting because of the armour that completely covered them). This gives us a visual image of personal power. The difficult thing is to give up that power, the lance, and offer ourselves. It gives the other party the choice to exercise their power of love by not killing you or their love of power by killing you.

In *Parzival* by Wolfram von Eschenbach we read of the knights fighting for the women's favours. By demonstrating their skill with the lance, they believe they capture the heart of a lady. At the end of the book, the women prevent them from fighting, saying *that* is the only way to win their love. The power of love overcomes the power of the sword — to quote a well-known passage, we can "turn swords into ploughshares".[26]

So what is this power of love? First we dance it as a feeling of community in a women's dance from Macedonia which is done in a front basket-weave handhold, in which we open our arms out and hold the hand of the person next door but one. It is a slow dance — so simple, so gentle and yet so powerful. We all have to move together, the handhold demands it. Of necessity we take small, considerate steps, moving rhythmically as one unit. This is the power that love has to bring us together as a gentle, persistent force for good in the world.

A dance choreographed to a South American tune gives a very different side to this power of love. It is exuberant, it celebrates life. We use it here to demonstrate the sheer joy of being together. It leaves us feeling

---

25. *The Symbolic Meaning of the Story of King Arthur* (King Arthur's Hall, Tintagel) p.6.
26. *The Bible*, Isaiah, chapter 2, verse 4.

good about ourselves, our companions and the whole of life. This love of life is what we must foster to bring love to all corners of the world. We can change our own perspective on life: life is what we make it. Even when we are going through difficult times we can change our outlook by treating every challenge as a means of growth. It then becomes something to celebrate rather than to rail against.

The power of love is in its giving and receiving: it is interesting to consider that someone who gives all the time and finds it impossible to receive can really be quite selfish. We have to allow others to give to us: the exchange is what gives love its power. We illustrate this with one of the Dances of Universal Peace: in these the group makes its own music by singing a song at the same time as doing the movements with the feet and the hands. The words of this one are:

> From you I receive
> To you I give
> Together we share
> By this we live.

So simple yet what truth they reveal. We face a partner and to the first line of the song extend our hands to the other person and draw them back towards us in receipt of their 'gift'. To the second line we do the reverse and give them a 'gift'. We then place our right hand on the other person's heart centre while our left hand covers their hand on our heart as we sing the third line. A deep and powerful contact is made. As the song ends we put our hands together in the prayer/namaste position which is an acknowledgement of the divinity within the other: we bow to our partner. Then we move on and the process is repeated to the next person round the circle.

I have seen people in tears doing this dance. Its simplicity is moving; the genuineness and acceptance that is demonstrated is unusual in our normal lives. Here we find these qualities lovingly and powerfully given and received. We are at one with ourselves and each other and once again the power of love is experienced.

In Kore we find another aspect of this: it is the power of love to unite a group, to give them a common purpose. Kore is another name for Persephone. Very briefly, in Greek mythology Persephone was captured by the King of the Underworld to be his bride. Persephone's mother, Demeter, the Goddess of the corn, was devastated when she could not find her daughter. She declared that the Earth would be barren until Persephone was safely back home. She wandered the length and breadth of the Earth, which was indeed barren. Eventually she learned of

Persephone's fate and pleaded with the King of the Underworld to set her free. He agreed on condition that she did not eat anything on her journey out of Hades. He cunningly dropped pomegranate seeds in her path and she ate six of them: he declared that she must return to be with him for one month for every seed consumed. That is why we have six months of summer and six of winter!

The story in itself demonstrates the power that love has. Demeter's love was strong enough to stop the Earth being fruitful. Even the King of the Underworld's love caused him to ensure that his beloved returned to him for part of the year. The power of the dance is in the movements we all do together, uniting us in creating a beautiful form. During the dance our hands are in continuous motion: in the first three steps we move forwards slowly bringing up the hands to shoulder height; in the second three we turn to move backwards and the hands reach a point behind us: then we move into the centre as the hands lift right up above us; as we move out again the hands return to our sides. As soon as the hands reach one extreme position, they start their journey towards the next: the motion is unhurried and unforceful — we do not push our neighbour into submission, it is an allowing, an acceptance. The power of this unity of purpose in such a gentle dance is quite incredible.

Power of love in silence

When we come to the sharing after these dances I have known the group to just sit in silence for a long while. By this time they are feeling comfortable with each other, there is no need to speak, they just want to absorb the experience, take it into themselves and consider how it might change their own lives. Perhaps this is another demonstration of the power of love. We find it difficult to be at peace with ourselves and others to the extent that we can be quiet. Yet at the end of a joint experience of this sort it seems natural and comfortable.

The workshop is drawing to a close and we join in a visualisation which leads us to a part of the world where the power of love is needed. We reflect on how the power of love may affect the lives of the people there in a clear and practical way. The visualisation ends with the words:

> Hold your image clearly in your mind and allow your heart to feel an intense will that it should take form. Let your heartfelt will build and, at the point of maximum intensity, send your idea, your image, your thought out into the world with direction and intent. Let it go. Do not cling to it.

Is this the essence of the power of love: that we feel another's need, we give with love and then let go, not dependent on outcomes or gratitude?

We conclude with a meditation dance to a piece by Bach. There is only one basic step which is repeated in different directions. In between we stand and raise our arms above our heads, then slowly lower them again. As I have been writing this chapter I have been struck by how many dances we use in this workshop which involve raising the arms: it is a position in which the heart is truly open. This is the essence of the power of love — its openness, its vulnerability. So often we are confronted by paradox: it is true that love is strong because it is vulnerable.

Taking it out to the world

I would like to conclude by quoting from the Dalai Lama's address to the Earth Summit in Rio de Janeiro (UNCED) in 1992.

> Whether we like it or not, we have all been born on this earth as part of one great family, rich or poor, educated or uneducated, belonging to one nation, religion, ideology or another, ultimately each of us is just a human being like everyone else. We all desire happiness and do not want suffering. Furthermore, each of us has the same right to pursue happiness and avoid suffering. When you recognise that all beings are equal in this respect, you automatically feel empathy and closeness to them. Out of this, in turn, comes a genuine sense of universal responsibility — the wish to actively help others overcome their problems.

Of course, this sort of compassion is, by nature, peaceful and gentle, but it is also very powerful. It is the true sign of inner strength. We do not need to become religious, nor do we need to believe in an ideology. All that is necessary is for each of us to develop our good human qualities.

Epilogue

Richard and Lynn

We end where we began — in Poland. It is the summer of 1997. The south of the country is devastated by major flooding. Żegiestów, the lovely little spa town where this book was conceived, is under floodwater. It is hard to imagine. Our hearts go out as we witness the pain of our friends. The news each evening shows the scale of the destruction — it is overwhelming. Evening dance sessions are delayed until after the news bulletin. We are brought up short and life is put into some kind of proportion.

We are running 'Dancing the Sevenfold Energies of Life' over a period of seven days — one of our dreams has come true. One occasion stands out: dancing Nigun Shel Yossi, a fast partner dance from Israel. Lynn is teaching from the outside of the circle because on the first day she fell down some steps and damaged both her feet! Without her in the circle, the dancers are struggling to learn the movements, confused as to which direction they should be travelling, and the whole thing seems to be turning into chaos.

"Just close your eyes for a moment and be still," Lynn says, "Imagine yourself doing the dance. See the direction in which you are travelling. Visualise doing the steps perfectly." A pause while the group pictures the scene. "OK, now let's do it!"

The result is electrifying; Lynn is almost reduced to tears watching the beauty of the dance and the miracle that has occurred. "That was beautiful," she exclaims with a lump in her throat. Andrzej comes over with a big white handkerchief! They have done it — for themselves, for each other and for Lynn.

The qualities of the Seven Rays become alive: a will and determination to do the dance; a bond of love between the dancers; tremendous activity and adaptation within the dance; beauty emerging, as harmony is found amidst confusion; mindfulness of the steps, direction and pattern; enthusiastic devotion to the dream of getting this one right; and the final achievement of coming together in rhythmic order.

We are with people who are facing disaster on a national scale. They discover, through the dance, qualities they will need in the days and months ahead. We all need these qualities in our lives as we face our challenges and opportunities. We all share in the dance of life, struggling with the steps and direction. We all need that moment of stillness in which to dream and visualise our way forward. Then we can believe that the dream can come true.

With self awareness we dance the sevenfold circle.

Appendices

by Lynn and Richard

Reflections for the Future

We have discovered over the years during which we have been running the *Self Awareness in Dance* workshops that this way of working lends itself to a wide variety of themes. Probably there is no end to the diverse topics that can be set to dance. When we started out we only had the one workshop in view: now we find ourselves always ready to explore new possibilities. We are also exploring the idea of designing workshops for groups around particular themes. It seems to be a natural development.

Sacred Geometry — Dancing the Maze and the Spiral

This idea came from a suggestion by a numerologist friend who was looking for a theme to work with in dance. Mazes and labyrinths were traditionally symbolic paths of transformation that individuals trod in order to confront themselves or to journey towards the revelation of greater light.

Anyone who has trodden a carefully laid out maze will know the uplifting effect it can bestow. A few years back we walked the turf maze on St Catherine's Hill in Winchester. It is not really very big and yet it certainly took us around 20 minutes to walk to the centre. You are compelled into a state of mindfulness as you move along the path. The first thing that happens is that you move sharply towards the centre. Can it be that simple? No! Immediately you are taken back out to the circumference and so begins the long and winding journey. Then, a great many steps later and when you are convinced you have trodden every possible twist and turn of the path, and are sure that somehow there is no route to the centre, you suddenly take a sharp turn and there you are, journey's end. Well, halfway at least because you cannot reach the centre of a maze or labyrinth and simply step out of it. The path has to be retraced.

It is a very different experience on the way out. The pace changes, and shifts in mood can be experienced. Sometimes there can seem to be a greater urgency and yet not in the sense of it being a hurry to get out, rather a certain purposefulness seems to pervade your attitude. On finally reaching the entrance once again the hope is that you arrive back at the start with more than you left with.

There are many dances that require us to move in spiral or labyrinthine form. The workshop is a way for participants to dance their way into themselves, into the light, and into the discovery of human and spiritual potential.

Dancing into Wellness

During 1996 we spent a weekend at Findhorn participating in a 'Medical Marriage' conference that brought together health-care professionals from the orthodox and complementary fields. We were there to run a mini-workshop on the theme 'From the Love of Power to the Power of Love', which proved to be extremely popular.

Another participant, Patch Adams, a medical doctor and clown from the USA, had been talking on the theme of 'wellness', a topic very close to his own heart and one that we found inspirational. How rarely do we actually talk or think in terms of 'wellness'? The beauty of the word is that it is not limited to health and all the associations that this word carries with it. Wellness is more than health, it embraces the social, cultural, familial and the spiritual, and every other facet of the human experience.

So we have found ourselves pondering on a day of 'Dancing into Wellness'. We certainly know many dances that can help us to feel well. Indeed, it seems to me that at the heart of wellness is the ability to be human and Sacred Circle Dance certainly encourages this. We hope it will not be too long before it is on our programme.

Experiencing Empathy in Dance

In Sacred Circle Dance people develop sensitivity towards each other. There has to be negotiation and co-operation in the circle in order for the collective movement to occur. We have to be mindful of the people on either side and may need to cultivate sensitivity to their style of dance. It may be quite different from our own, it may be very similar; we do not know until we share the dance experience together. Empathy is important and potent in co-operative movement. As the circle moves we each take our space and our own movements with us on a journey, hand in hand with others. We form a relationship with the people on either side, for without a firm and secure connection with them we can isolate ourselves from the group experience.

It may simply be about how firmly we hold hands, or how freely (or not) our arms move in rhythm with the music. It could be that we need to adjust our speed to those around us, or they need to adjust to us! The fact remains, however, that when people are seeking to move together, whether in dance or in a therapeutic relationship, or in any other aspect of life, empathy with the other person or persons is required. Dance encourages us in effect to sacrifice our own interests in the greater purpose of creating a group experience.

'Experiencing Empathy in Dance' in the context of therapeutic groups and training offers not only a safe space for us to develop sensitivity to those around us, but also brings to light those petty irritations and hindrances within our natures that block us from giving ourselves to the spirit of relationship.

Dancing into the love conditions

After developing the idea of exploring empathy through dance we began to think of ways in which we could apply dance to Carl Rogers' core conditions which include congruence and unconditional positive regard as well. These three qualities, when present in a therapeutic relationship, enhance the possibility of personal growth.

How do we achieve this? We have already indicated how dance can enable us to experience empathy with each other and the dance form itself. There are dances in which we are required to move individually, affording us the opportunity to explore our individual self-expression. We have a little more space in which to work and in which to be ourselves. This can allow us to be a little more free, an opportunity to experience ourselves without so much concern for what is happening with the people in the rest of the circle.

Unconditional positive regard is emphasised through dances that involve one-to-one interaction. There are many partner-dances, or dances that involve a chain so that we move from partner to partner. We use dances that encourage eye contact and co-ordinated interaction. It provides us with an opportunity to meet and greet people in relationship. It is a safe place to do this, contained by the rhythm and form of the dance. It can be an incredibly powerful experience to give and receive unconditional positive regard.

A lot of counselling and psychotherapy is word-based. In the dance there is no need for words. Fresh forms of communication open up. New sensitivities emerge as we touch and are touched psychologically through unconditional relationship with another person.

The Dance of Life

Perhaps the most challenging of themes for a workshop is life itself. Yet we feel that dance can play a vital role in helping us acknowledge what life and the process of living means to us. What is life? What does it feel like to be alive? What is this something that we call living that some find so compelling and vital, yet others find quite impossible to face? This workshop is planned specifically to explore life in its many facets and to celebrate what it has brought to us. We look at creativity and expression through movement, the cycles of nature, human relationship and interaction. It is an immense topic and yet it is perhaps the most fundamental of all themes.

Is there a 'One Life'? What do we mean by this? What relevance does the idea have for human living? These are enormous questions that we do not usually stop and reflect on. We can be so full of 'busy-ness' that we fail to extend our horizon beyond the immediate needs. We hope that in 'The Dance of Life' we can change this and create an opportunity, if you like, to stop our personal world for a moment and to take a look around ourselves, to explore and to learn.

Perhaps, most important, is to give ourselves time to wonder, to wonder at the immensity, the beauty, the fragility and the power of life. Do we ever stop to wonder, looking at the night sky or the delicate and intricate shapes of creation? To wonder is to regain a sense of awe-struck humility. We are somehow put in our place in the scheme of things, no longer inflating our own self-importance, rather affirming the small part that we play within the great process that we call life.

Is life a subject for scientific study or artistic exploration? Some would say it is an either/or choice. Yet surely it is both that we need: a science of life and an art of living.

Life really is a dance, for a dance encompasses movement, relation-ship, energy, direction, change, creativity — the list is endless. To spend a day or a weekend to simply open our hearts and our minds (and, of course, our bodies) to this process of being will bring us all closer to our true selves and our potential to live life to the full. In this day we honour the personal and the spiritual, considering the human experience within the context of spiritual growth.

Of course, at the end of the day we each have to return to our per-sonal circles of life to face our own unique challenges and opportunities. This is inevitable. The workshop is not a means of escape but a way of gaining strength so that we can return renewed and refreshed, our hopes and ideals given a boost, and with our intention to live life and to love life strengthened.

Preparing for the New Millennium

Once again a theme emerged out of a workshop experience. We were asked if we were planning anything special for the millennium celebra-tions. No ... but wait a minute, are we really prepared for the new millennium? Could we use dance to explore this particular transition which is going to affect everyone on the planet? What do people think and feel about the year 2000 and beyond? Do we really have much op-portunity to share our ideas and to offer each other support and encouragement?

This workshop is now being offered and we will be providing an opportunity for participants to explore this major transition within the life of humanity. We will give people the chance to really look at what it means to them: their hopes and their fears, their vision for the future. We will also offer the opportunity for people to consider how they wish to celebrate the millennium and empower them to make it happen. Just writing about this workshop arouses great excitement in us. It seems so right, so appropriate and so timely.

Other ideas

We see huge scope for using dance in many areas of human activity and relationship. The following are some of the ideas that we are keen to develop. If you have experience in any of these areas we are interested in exploring what we can offer.

Counselling, psychotherapy and psychology

We would like to integrate our workshops into psychology courses, and counselling and psychotherapy training. In particular, 'Dancing the Sevenfold Energies of Life' would provide a valuable context for people seeking to develop greater self-awareness, and would certainly draw out material for discussion and further work. At any time in such a course it would be a useful learning tool: at the beginning people would gain personal insight; later on a repeat or refresher would stimulate further understanding of themselves and others; at the end of a group process it would be a powerful ritual — by this time the dances are familiar and participants would be able to experience them in a new and powerful way.

We do not describe what we do as dance therapy because this is not what it is. Dance therapy is a specific discipline. However, our approach is therapeutic and can have a healing effect on those who participate.

Any discipline which requires human-to-human interaction, and particularly those in which this provides the basis for therapeutic change, could benefit from what we offer. To relate to others in a manner that is healing and helpful requires us to understand ourselves, to be in touch with how we relate to others and to feel freed up to be our human self with our clients.

Management training and teambuilding

People who are working together towards a common goal and for whom inter- and intra-personal relationships are important, would benefit from Sacred Circle Dance. Staff in medical settings, for instance, or other emergency services, even sports teams, could gain a great deal from the experience of community dance. As we will see in the next chapter, where we describe our *Unity in Diversity* teambuilding initiative, the scope for bringing teams together symbolically and in reality through Sacred Circle Dance is exciting and full of innovative potential.

Schools and young people

There is great scope for working with children and young people. Perhaps Sacred Circle Dance could be introduced into schools. We both remember country dancing from our primary school days. Maybe we could help children and young people to gain insight into their own natures through dance? Certainly it would contribute to co-ordination and spatial-awareness skills. Added to this would be experiences in co-operation and negotiation, in achieving goals in a non-competitive environment and in taking responsibility for their own experiences and the effect that they have on those around them.

It would also offer alternative dancing experience to the seemingly all-pervasive disco and club scene. This would enable young people to widen their horizons. There would be scope for them to engage with their own feelings in a safe and supportive environment, to celebrate and to gain insight into themselves. This, then, provides them with a resource for making choices and decisions.

It would expose them to other cultures and traditions, enriching their educational experience. Imagine what a child could learn by being taken round the world in dance.

Peace-building

We feel that these dances could be introduced specifically as a peace-building exercise for community representatives to come together, share common experiences and establish lines of human-to-human communication. This could be organised locally by community groups in any setting. Yet it could extend beyond this. It may seem far-fetched, but why should not the United Nations adopt dance as a strategy for peace-building? Or The Commonwealth? Or the European Union? Sometimes we can communicate a great deal more through shared experience than through the words of diplomatic negotiation.

Human-to-human contact that leaves us smiling and appreciating the qualities and the pleasure of others is the basis for community and co-operative living. If we can find a way to put aside our differences and conflicts in the joy and excitement of the dance, and as a result we experience something good, positive and heartfelt in ourselves, then we know what is possible in our communities. We often live on the surface, acting and reacting, living out habits of relating, of fearing, of hating, passed down from generation to generation. We can only stop this by giving ourselves the opportunity to experience something new, something more real in our hearts in human-to-human interaction. Sacred Circle Dance can provide a basis for peaceful co-existence.

Stress management

There is an important role for Sacred Circle Dance in stress management. The experience of the dance can be energising and renewing. It can encourage relaxation and, when coupled with visualisation exercises, helps people to unwind and enables them to find a more serene place within themselves. Let us put fun into stress management. We sincerely believe that regular Sacred Circle Dance in teams would generate a community sense that would ensure that the group was far more self-supporting, with its members much more sensitive to each other's needs.

We seem to be forever hearing of stress and its effects. Do we ever stop to question why this is? What is it about our society that induces the need for stress management? Stress can be simplified to two areas:

- The effect of doing or experiencing that which you do not want to do or to experience.
- The effect of having to do too much of what you want to do or to experience.

Sacred Circle Dance is so different from our usual routine that we can break free for a short space of time and gain a fresh perspective on our situation. We can take a moment to connect with our own needs and, by distancing ourselves from the demands being placed on us, re-evaluate and reformulate our schedules.

Conclusion

No doubt there are many other areas in which *Self Awareness in Dance* would find a useful role. Whilst we have our own ideas, we are always looking for new opportunities, and welcome discussion with anyone who has a concept or a setting in which to experiment. Dance is a universal language.

Unity in Diversity Teambuilding

Another development that emerged out of our stay at the Findhorn Community in 1996 was the idea of using some of our themes specifically for the purpose of teambuilding. It began to take off whilst sitting in a café on the Isle of Skye and, as is so often the case, we had not sat down with the intention of thinking about this. It simply began to bubble in our minds and soon the soup and crusty roll was sharing the table with bits of paper and scribbled ideas!

Following our mini-workshop at the Medical Marriage conference, one participant commented wistfully "I wish some of my managers could experience this kind of thing". It had sown a seed in our minds. At the end of the Conference we were asked to write down what intention we would be taking away with us. We were then offered an opportunity to share it with everyone else. Richard, microphone in hand, declared "I want to bring Sacred Circle Dance into the world of corporate teambuilding". A cheer went up from the audience; when it had died down, he continued "But I haven't told Lynn yet!" Lynn quickly grabbed the microphone and announced "That was exactly what I wrote down too". Another cheer!

The first thing that became clear to us, as we sat looking out over the Skye coastline, watching the scene before us shift and change in the light, was the idea of calling it *Unity in Diversity*. We have both felt that this phrase carried a lot of meaning and significance for our time. So much of our diversity is not celebrated and very often difference is regarded as a threat to be fought against rather than to be shared as an enriching experience for everyone. We also feel that within us there is scope to discover common ground, a centre from which we can create a unity of spirit and purpose. The little-used word 'unanimity' is one that we would like to see brought back into more common usage, reflecting its true meaning which is 'unity of Soul'.

Philosophy of teamwork

We found ourselves considering what the philosophy of *Unity in Diversity* teambuilding might be. The ideas soon began to flow, the whole concept seemed to be taking on a life of its own and the next few days involved a lot more scribbling on pieces of paper. One of the first things that struck us was that we could explore team dynamics, roles and responsibilities from the angle of the Seven Rays. The members of the team will express these energies in their own individual and unique ways. We could bring this out into the open, helping them to appreciate their own, and each other's, strengths and potentials. We could enable teams to consciously use these energies to help them be more effective in their roles.

We see a team as a circle. Individual members have their own position in relation to the others and have contact through their colleagues with the whole. For a team to function at its maximum potential, each member's qualities and strengths must be acknowledged and valued. The strength of the team as a whole lies in bringing together these individual qualities in unanimity of purpose.

As in music, harmony is achieved by sounding different notes in a rhythmic relationship. Following this analogy, the work of the team becomes a rhythmic movement in circular form with commonality of purpose: this is empowering and rewarding. The circle represents wholeness and completeness. Every team member is essential in creating that cohesion and yet has a unique task to perform.

The circle becomes a living and moving metaphor for the unity of the team. The movement of each individual member reflects his/her personal style within the team. Bringing these together in a context which is free of the associations of the daily work routine, a new dynamic of human interaction emerges, to be harnessed and applied to particular tasks, goals and responsibilities.

The experience of the dance is total, a team creation in which each has played his/her part. We feel good, we feel empowered, we feel ready to face the next challenge. This can be seen as a microcosm of the fully functional team in the work environment.

So what is a team and how can it function?

Let us explore some of these ideas in a little more detail. First, our philosophy of teams is rooted in the idea that we are each unique individuals with our own diverse talent and potential. We need to recognise what these are, and, for the manager, the task is to play to an employee's strengths. Through the experience of the dance, individuals can gain insight into their strengths, into their natural ways of functioning. They can also gain a better appreciation of how their colleagues function.

This helps to break down barriers and enables them to see a little more of the whole person with whom they work. So often the office environment is a single-track setting which blocks this process from occurring. We believe strongly that teams are far more effective when the individuals that comprise them are able to bring more of their whole self into the team, rather than one aspect of themselves. The effect of this is a much fuller relationship between people, which increases the scope and the depth of co-operation, and the team spirit. In the context of the Seven Rays, knowing who is most effective at expressing a particular energy could be invaluable, for instance, in project management. Also, having a diverse range of Ray types within a team may enrich its creative potential and produce opportunities for cross-fertilisation of ideas and perspectives.

People often use this phrase 'team spirit' and it is worth considering just what it is. Anyone who has worked in or with groups will appreciate how often in discussion 'the group' is talked about, almost as if it has become an identity in and of itself. "The group feels this ...", "the group cannot cope with that ....", "the group has no direction". The group only exists because a set of individuals has come together in relationship to pursue a particular task. The group then becomes a product of three things:

- The individuals
- The relationships between the individuals
- The task

This is basic and obvious, but it is often important to simplify things in order to build from a firm foundation.

The individuals

Each person is unique, having his or her own skills and motivation to be part of the enterprise. Each individual will have certain expectations and a whole stream of experiences that have contributed to shaping them to be the way they are. Yet in many teams, much of this is invisible or not known by managers. Time has not been taken to get to know the person. We call people individuals but do we treat them as such? Do we consciously seek to honour their individuality, or do they get clumped together in our minds, or categorised as 'a this' or 'a that' type and treated accordingly (though not necessarily appropriately). Our experience as individuals in work settings is simple: when honoured as a person, as an individual with a unique set of experiences, we find ourselves more motivated and loyal towards the team or the organisation.

We are moving beyond the concept that work is something we have to do grudgingly, and leisure is what we do for ourselves. The fully-functional person is looking for fulfilment in all aspects of his or her life.

Whilst there is an economic need for work in strictly financial terms, there is also a human need to be creative and to co-operate with others, to face challenges individually and collectively, and to be able to look back and feel a sense of pride and well-being at a task done well.

It is also interesting to note that in community circle dance, when the circle moves off-centre each individual has the power and potential to bring it back into balance. However, if nobody takes responsibility but assumes that someone else will do it, the circle may continue to move further away from the centre. It reinforces awareness that, for a team to function in balanced relationship and centred around its task, each individual has to take responsibility for maintaining this and has power to achieve it (Figures 27 and 28).

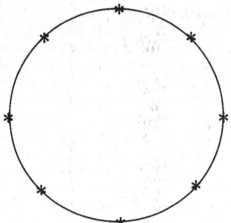

Figure 27.
Circle in balance

In Figure 27 we have a circle, centred and in balance. Each individual is in the right place and in right relationship with the rest of the circle and the centre (which could represent the task).

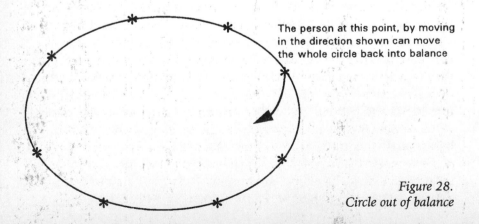

The person at this point, by moving in the direction shown can move the whole circle back into balance

Figure 28.
Circle out of balance

In Figure 28 the circle is distorted and off-centre. This is because the individuals are out of balance and are not pulling together equally. Nobody is taking responsibility for bringing the circle (team) back into a balanced position. However, one person can give a lead as indicated and, if there is co-operation, the circle can move back to its former position. The ability of an individual to influence the whole circle (or team) is based on the fact of relationship between the individuals and with the common task. When there is connection, one person can generate movement, so long as the whole team understands the task and the direction in which it is seeking to travel.

The relationships

The relationships that we have with our colleagues, and with managers, are a crucial part of a team. We may talk a lot about the importance of the individual, but unless each individual is relating well with the rest of the team, individual potential can be lost. Do we really give much thought to the nature of our working relationships? Are we clear on where our boundaries are, where our role and responsibility touch those of a colleague? It is worth considering who we work with most in our own settings; who we feel comfortable with and who we do not; and how this affects our interactions with other people. Do we avoid colleagues that we need to communicate with for effective working? Do we lean more towards others who may have less expertise but whom we like more and find more approachable?

We often hear the phrase "do not mix business and pleasure". Oh dear, must business therefore gain the distinction of being unpleasurable? Teams by their nature are social groups that involve complex relationships. Once we begin to try to bring more of ourselves into the team relationship, we are more likely to be treated as a complete person and we are going to find the experience more pleasurable and fulfilling.

In settings outside the normal working environment such as the dancing circle, there is a much greater opportunity for habitual reactions that have developed in the workplace to stand out more clearly for what they are, because they will be seen to be inappropriate. We get locked into habits and patterns and ways of acting, reacting and interacting in relationships. These patterns become normalised for us when continued over time, to the point that they feel natural, and indeed may even become unconscious. For the dancing circle to work, there is a requirement for negotiation and co-operation, for spatial awareness and for personal adjustment to the group movement and process.

The task

In the workshop the task is to perform a dance as a group, allowing each individual to express themselves freely yet to honour each other's expression. In the world of work it may be a specific project that has brought a team of individuals together in relationship. What is crucially important is that the task becomes central. Added to this, there has to be clarity as to each person's role and responsibility, and inter-personal appreciation of each other's qualities and skills. But the task is paramount because, in the final analysis, it is the team's *raison d'être*.

For the team to fulfil its purpose, the defined task has to be completed efficiently and effectively, with everyone contributing their specialist skills in co-operation with one another. All need to feel part of the process and therefore able to own their contribution and the final goal when it is reached. As the individuals need to understand the relationships they have with each other within the process, so they need to understand how their creativity has contributed to the final achieved goal. Everyone's effort will have been necessary and therefore each can take pride in their contribution. If someone's contribution has truly been unnecessary then the team was put together inefficiently, but that is another subject.

We can consider the triplicity of task, relationship and individual from the perspective of the Seven Rays, described earlier. There is a correspondence between the energy of Will or Power and the *task*; the energy of Love-Wisdom and the *relationship* that forms the team; the energy of Active Intelligence and the *individuals* whose creativity enables the team to achieve its task. This can be represented diagrammatically (Figure 29).

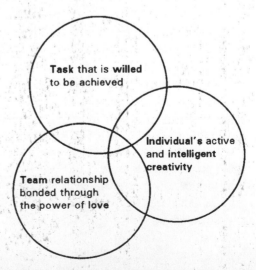

Figure 29.
Triplicity of function and energy

The circles could also be seen not simply overlapping but rather overlaid on each other. The problem with any model of this kind is that the complexity of the system gets lost in the form of the representation. The model is not the reality. We are in truth looking at a complex system of relationships, functions and processes in which all three elements interact in a kind of continuum, each affecting the others.

So another way of looking at it is to create a circle with all three located on the circumference (Figure 30). In this model of the team, each team function interconnects directly with the others, as well as via the third function.

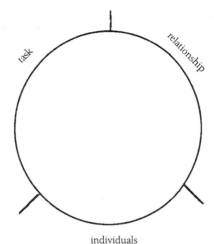

Figure 30.
The team continuum

Here task, relationship and individuals are brought together in a single circle, a continuum of connection to be held in balance. This requires all three facets of the team to be in touch with each other. Here we have the 'team circle' represented symbolically.

In the final analysis, all creative endeavour begins with an idea. If we can adjust our thinking about what a team is and how it functions, we can reshape the creative process, and ensure that the task is completed effectively and efficiently. Within this process the team members involved are enabled to feel fulfilled and honoured as individuals, and to experience a quality of co-operative relationship that has application within the wider human society.

Index

A

Arcane School 23–24
Armenia 67
art of living 219
Arthurian legends 209
astral plane, children 90
astrology, esoteric 123

B

Bailey, Alice 22, 76, 133
balance 132
beliefs, questioning 11
Besant, Annie 22
Blavatsky, Madame 21, 22
blocks, resolving 100
Brazil 107
Britain 104
Bulgaria 66–67

C

candle 51, 67
    symbolism of 49
channelling 19
children, sensitivity of 87
China 108
Christ 112
    crosses 159
    teachings of 11
Christmas 175–176
circle
    centre 114
    squaring the 159, 161
    symbolism 154
coincidence 13–14, 15, 30, 62, 200
colour
    healing 98
    perception 97–98
community, global 127

complements 166
connectedness 29, 47, 70
    across time 22
conscious evolution 23
consciousness 86, 94, 124
    group 139
    time 95
costume 71
counselling 26–27
crisis
    of expression 89
    of opportunity 89
cross 125, 140
    and circle 51
    symbolism 154
cycle
    life 54
    of change 195
    seasons 158
    zodiac 158
cycles of time 178

D

Dalai Lama 212
dance, of life 114
de Chardin, Teilhard 22
desirelessness 126
diversity 183
duality 126, 168, 179, 198

E

egg
    Easter 152
    symbolism 152
Eire 58–59
Emerson, Ralph Waldo 22
empathy 64, 212, 217
evolution 93

F

Findhorn 11, 40
Former Yugoslavia 68–69
Fountain International 46
France 106

G

Gandhi 50
Geldof, Bob 25
Germany 106
glamour 100, 125
golden mean 162
Goldsmith, Joel 22
goodwill 186–187, 188
Great Invocation 187
Greece 69–70
group work 36–38
growth 111

H

harmony 18–19
heart 112, 170
    awakening 139
hurt, effect of 25

I

initiation 135–136
intuition 130
Israel 61–63, 71–73
Iran 73
Italy 107
Itteringham Mill 22

J

Jung, Carl 22

K

karma 21, 89
knowledge 146
Krishnamurti 22

L

labyrinth 126, 215
life-cycle 85
    Jung 157
    Rays 90
    stages 87–90
Live Aid 25
love 24, 110–112
Lovelock, James 25
Lucis Trust 24–25

M

Macedonia 70–71
mandala 51, 163
meditation 11, 51
    study and service 23–24
mid-life 86, 90
mirror-image 56
moment, power of 26
muscle memory 48

N

Neville, Derek 22

O

opposites 166

P

pain 111
Paine, Thomas 22
paradox 52, 54, 177, 185, 198, 212
peace 134, 221
pentagram 162
Person-Centred Approach
    spirituality 27–28
personal growth 180
personality 87, 129
Poland 5, 60–61, 63
psychology, esoteric 89

R

Ramacharaka, Yogi

Ray
    definition 76
    emotional 78
    mental 78
    personality 79
    physical 78
    Soul 79
Rays
    groups 83
    nations 103
    strengths/weaknesses 81
    triplicity 85
rebirth 88, 123, 125
relationship 25, 33, 99, 217
    Rays 1 and 2 81
responsibility 105, 111, 136
Rogers, Carl 22, 217
Romania 65–66
Russia 68, 105

S

Sacred Circle Dance
    and sacred space 42
    and Seven Rays 32, 35
    and spirituality 47
    and unanimity 48
    animals 52
    as a language 58–64
    as a mirror 38
    community 41
    effects 10, 17, 20
    first encounter 11
    first group 14
    origins of 40–47
    with children 16
sacred space, creating 42–47
Savill Gardens 98
science of life 219
separateness 127, 133
service 25, 88, 111, 130, 138
Seven Rays
    tetrahedron 85

    and Sacred Circle Dance 32, 35
sevenfold circle 120
shadow 43, 57
silence 53, 211
solar plexus 170
Soul 86, 87, 111
    expression through service 24
    true essence 21
Soul-centred psychology 28
Spangler, David 22
spiral 30, 55, 94, 170, 172
Spirit 176
spiritual
    growth 30
    path 24
spirituality 14, 34, 47, 49, 180
spontaneity 177, 180
stability, need for 21
stress 222
swastika 156
symbolism 53

T

teambuilding 223
time 22, 54
    continuum 34
    elastic 95
timing 95, 181
transcendence 172
transition 106
trust 33–34
truth, finding our own 11, 18–19, 21

U

UNCED 107, 212
universality 88
USA 104

W

wellness 216
wisdom 146
Wosien, Bernhard 40

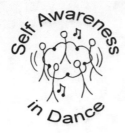

Lynn Frances and Richard Bryant-Jefferies
can be contacted at
The Hart Centre
2 Harts Gardens
Guildford
Surrey GU2 6QA
email lynnrichard@hartcentre.demon.co.uk
url http://www.hartcentre.demon.co.uk

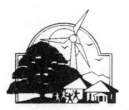

The Findhorn Community
can be contacted at
Findhorn Foundation
The Park
Findhorn
Forres IV36 0TZ
tel 01309 690311
fax 01309 691301
email reception@findhorn.org
url http://www.findhorn.org

Findhorn Press presents the Spirit of Dance collection:

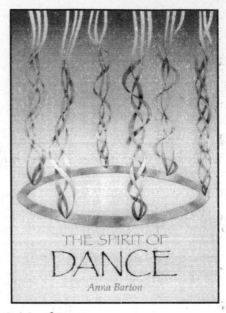

Part 1 — The Spirit of Dance
- booklet 28-pp ISBN 0-905249-71-2 £3.50/us$5.50
- audio-cassette £7.00/us$10.00
- video-cassette (PAL format only) £13.99

Part 2 — The Spirit of Dance: the Next Steps
- booklet 32-pp ISBN 0-905249-82-8 £3.95/us$6.00
- audio-cassette £7.00/us$10.00

For any of the above or a complete book and music catalogue,
please contact:

Findhorn Press
The Press Building
The Park
Findhorn
Forres IV36 0TZ
Scotland
tel 01309 690582
fax 01309 690036

Findhorn Press
P. O. Box 13939
Tallahassee
Florida 32317-3939
USA

email thierry@findhorn.org
url http://www.findhorn.org/findhornpress/